A Peace of Hope

Finding Inner Peace and
Healing Through Stage IV Cancer

Brittney Beadle

ISBN: 979-8-218-28920-1

In the pages that follow, I invite you to join me on an intimate healing journey, captured through the lens of personal journal entries of my first four years living with metastatic breast cancer.

Finding my inner peace was pivotal for me. No matter how bad things seemed to get I knew as long as I had inner peace the uncertainty couldn't have power over me. I fell many times, but deep down I always knew I would have the power to rise again- and I did.

Hope, too, emerges throughout these pages - not just for me, but for you, the reader. My hope is that you'll find solace and inspiration- for you to know healing is always possible, no matter how dire the circumstances may seem. We all have the power within us, awaiting only our belief in it.

Here is A Peace of Hope from me to you.

Introduction

I grew up in a small town in Northeastern Pennsylvania, where I was free-spirited and danced to the beat of my own drum. I was raised by the most loving mother, who always encouraged me to be myself and to believe in magic and miracles. I like to believe I chose her before coming down to this earthly plane.

Growing up, I was close with my older brother, Jesse. He is three years older than me, but he and his friends never minded a rambunctious little girl tagging along with them. He wasn't a typical role model older sibling; he got in trouble a lot, but he helped guide me in his own special way. He was always the one to make the mistakes first, so I observed and learned from him. He would often say, "Don't be like me …" and then insert a fill-in-the-blank story. Thanks for taking one for the team, Jesse!

As a teenager, I had a bubbly personality, but on the inside, I felt sad and struggled with an eating disorder. I kept it as my little secret. In grade nine, I decided to enroll in my school's cyber school program. I worked during the day and then came home to do my schoolwork. I loved this setup because it gave me more independence. I also hated feeling "trapped" in one place. Being able to do my schoolwork from anywhere at any time meant I was free to travel with my mom whenever we wanted, which helped support my mental health.

I finally started healing from my inner wounds, only to be met with a new challenge. On a cold February night, I first found a lump in my breast. My boyfriend at the time saw it protruding from my right breast, almost as if it was begging to be found. I was freshly eighteen.

I told my mom, who then made me an appointment right away to get it checked. From there, I saw a breast specialist who ordered both an ultrasound and a mammogram. I remember this day vividly. It was a long day of waiting. As I sat in the waiting room, I was surrounded by posters about breast cancer, and there was a talk show on the TV mentioning the new *50 Shades of Grey* movie.

When I was done with all the tests for the day, the breast specialist said to me, "You do have a mass, but you are eighteen, and eighteen-year-olds don't get breast cancer," as she handed me a piece of paper that read "fibroadenoma" and sent me home.

When I arrived home, I gave the paper to my mom, who questioned it but decided to put her trust in the doctor. She still saved the paper, just in case. I think this was her intuition telling her something was wrong.

Three months passed by, and flowers were blooming, birds were singing, and the air was now warmer. I was in the tanning bed (I know, I cringe now too) when I noticed the lump had grown significantly, causing my nipple to invert. My biggest concern was that it looked ugly. *Oh, to be that naive.* My mom made me another appointment with the breast specialist, who took one look at it, and concern took over her face. I had yet another ultrasound and mammogram, both showing four new friends that had grown within that time. This time they biopsied one of the masses and told me they would call with the results. Little did I know the results would change my life forever.

The Disaster

Lotus flowers start life deep-rooted in muddy water. They survive in diverse climates, from scorching sun to freezing wind. They even survived the ice age. As long as their roots are kept in water or mud, they will survive.

Yet, sometimes they do die from natural disasters. In 1954 the flooding of the Yangtze River caused all the lotuses in the area to die, but when the water started to recede three years later, the lotus restored itself from the seeds that had been scattered before the flood.

Life, death, rebirth. The resilience of this flower is incredible. Through an ice age, mud, and even having roots ripped out from under them due to flooding, still they survived.

I am a lotus flower.

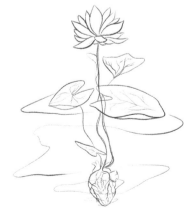

The Call

May 6th, 2015

Three months ago, a breast specialist said to me, "Eighteen-year-olds don't get breast cancer." I was at a check-up for a lump I had found in my right breast.

It was supposed to be nothing.

Yesterday, I went to the hospital to have an ultrasound, mammogram, and biopsy to check the same lump that had grown significantly and caused my nipple to invert.

It was supposed to be nothing.

That day started off like any other day. Actually, it started off better than any other day. I woke up feeling like sunshine, excited about life on your average Wednesday morning. I was sitting downstairs at my desk doing my online school work when I received the call to come into the hospital; my results were ready. I didn't think anything of it.

It was supposed to be nothing.

My mom couldn't come with me because she was at the chiropractor. She didn't think too much of it.

It was supposed to be nothing.

I called my boyfriend to come along and keep me company. With the windows rolled down, I felt the warm May breeze on my skin as we danced and sang to our favorite songs the entire way there.

It was supposed to be nothing.

When we arrived, a nurse brought my boyfriend and me into our own little room.

"Oh no, your mother couldn't make it here with you?" Her eyes were sad and conveyed concern.

"No," I responded with a confused look, wondering why she asked that.

It was supposed to be nothing.

A few minutes later, the breast specialist came into the room, sat down next to me, put her hand on my leg, and with regret in her voice, said, "The results showed you have breast cancer."

Numb.

After that, I went completely and utterly numb. The doctor was speaking, but I no longer heard what she was saying. All I could think was . . .

It was supposed to be nothing.

I looked up and saw my boyfriend with tears streaming down his face.

That is when it hit me. It wasn't nothing.

It was something.

At that moment, the first tear ran down my cheek. It quickly turned into a faucet that couldn't be turned off.

"I'll give you guys some time to process this. You should call your mom, and when she gets here, we will discuss more." These words came out of the doctor who told me three months ago, "Eighteen-year-olds don't get breast cancer."

It was something.

Mom broke down when I told her. I heard it in the crack of her voice when she said, "What?" in disbelief. She raced to the hospital but was so distraught she went to the wrong one first.

It was something.

When she arrived, she hugged me so tight. All three of us cried.

It was something.

After speaking to a few different doctors, we decided I would need a mastectomy.

It was something.

Today I am sad, confused, angry, and numb . . .

Tomorrow, I would be strong. Tomorrow I would pick up the pieces that broke that day.

I gave myself a day to feel absolutely everything.

It was something.

I knew deep in my soul I would be okay.

It was something.

Starry Night and Teary Eyes

Here we are
Lying on my favorite blanket, gazing at the stars
Into the infinite night sky
Not one word is said
Our hands intertwined
Heads resting gently together
But I still have no idea what is on your mind
I hope you stay
But it's okay if you don't
I'll understand
This is a lot on anyone
Especially the young like us
I never knew what my future would hold
Especially now
But I hope to see you in it

Overwhelmed
But Loved

So it begins was my first thought of the day after waking up with a phone call from a doctor who filled my week with nothing but appointments. Oncology, radiology, you name it, I had it. Cancerland was like being on a high-speed train. Things moved fast and felt completely overwhelming, but I was also so supported.

After meeting my new oncologist, I texted my boyfriend, Ben, and he darted out of class early to come to my rescue. I didn't ask him to, but he said he wanted to be there for me. He explained *we* are going through this, not just me. His words made my sunken spirit rise from despair.

It was starting to get warm here in NEPA, Northeastern Pennsylvania, so we sat on the stairs of my old wooden porch holding hands and discussing my appointments. I told him I would need chemotherapy and, most likely, radiation.

With tears in his eyes, Ben muttered, "I don't understand why this is happening to you. You are the most selfless, kind person I have ever met. It should have happened to me. I'm not even a nice person."

"Don't you dare say that," I said, shaking my head at him. Everyone in my family kept saying that to me. They all wished they could take it away, but as much as I wished I didn't have to go through this, I would never wish this upon them. I felt like this was happening for a reason, I didn't know what it was yet, but I could feel it.

My friends stopped by and surprised me with a care package today. I felt guilty because I wasn't the one to tell them. I didn't know how. I mean, how does one tell the people they love they have cancer? I gave my mom permission to write a Facebook post to let friends and family know and to ask for prayers. Maybe it wasn't the best way, but I didn't have the energy to have *that* conversation with everyone.

In the care package my friends brought was a journal so I could start documenting my journey. They wrote some uplifting messages for me inside, including this one by Elizabeth Edwards, "She stood in the storm, and when the wind did not blow her way, she adjusted her sails."

I was in awe of these amazing people I had in my life. You don't truly realize who is there for you until something like cancer comes along and tries to dismantle you. Some people step up, and some fade away.

Mastectomy

May 14th, 2015

I had to miss my senior prom today, but Amber, my best
friend, still came to visit me in the hospital. She was
all dressed up in a beautiful gown, hair curled, looking stunning. I was in a gown, too, a hospital gown with
scars on my chest where my nipples once were.

I never thought this would be my prom gown.

The before-

I woke up before sunrise to leave for the hospital at 5 o'clock.

I thought there would be more sadness about
losing my breasts, but that wasn't the case.

I felt like they were no longer mine. Cancer invaded my right
breast, and I didn't want to sit around and let the rest of my
body be at risk, so I am going to make my move while I can.

I'm ready to take back *my* body.

The after-

Confused, itchy, and tearful sums up
my post-surgery experience.

When I opened my eyes, I was in the recovery area.
I was separated off behind beige curtains.

I heard what sounded like an older man
sobbing on the right side of the curtains.

"Is it okay if I cry?" he asked one of the nurses.

I'm not sure why, but at that moment, I,
too, felt like I needed a good cry.

Once I started, I couldn't stop.

When I finally saw my family, Mom told me
it took much longer than expected.

My surgeon took his time to make sure
he got absolutely everything.

I'm grateful for him and all my incredible nurses.
Although I was completely unconscious, they said they
played some of my favorite songs during surgery.

I hope they know how much they make a difference.

Scars-

I'm having mixed feelings after seeing beneath
the bandages for the first time.

My stomach was in knots as my surgeon
started unwrapping my chest.

I gagged with disgust when I caught my
first glance of my new body.

I chose to delay reconstruction, so it was hard to
process shifting from a size DD to . . . nothing.

Just a flat chest with blood, bruising, and scars.

Oh, and two fluid-filled tubes hanging out of each side of me.

I have to trust that, over time, it will get
easier to look at myself again

and learn to love my body in its new form.

For now, I will focus on the bright side of it all.

They said they got everything, lymph nodes and all.

In my eyes, it's all worth it to be cancer free.

Metastatic

I am supposed to graduate high school in a few days.
I am supposed to be living out my dreams in Florida.
I am supposed to get married and have children.
I am supposed to help change the world.
I am supposed to live to be old and gray.
But ...
I am incurable with metastatic breast cancer.

Not Curable, But Treatable

June 12th, 2015

Due to my age, my oncologist felt more comfortable getting a second opinion on treatments. She set up an appointment for me at a top cancer hospital in New York. My mom, dad, grandfather, and boyfriend accompanied me. I really had the best crew by my side.

Walking into the appointment, I didn't know what the doctor—whom I was meeting for the first time—was going to drop on me.

I had a PET scan a little over a week ago and was starting to feel anxious about my results. My oncologist wasn't answering any of my phone calls, so I figured that meant it was clear, but I wanted confirmation. The second the doctor sat down, I blurted out, "How were my scan results?" I expected her to tell me they were nice and clean and nothing to worry about, but that is not what she said.

"You don't know?" she asked, tilting her head in disbelief.

"Know what?" I responded, very confused.

A concerned look arose on her face as she reached into the folder, took out my results, and pushed them toward me. "There are spots . . ." she began to say.

Instantly my heart sank. Everyone in the room with me fell silent.

"No, no! I think you have the wrong report. That is not hers," my mom said in denial.

The doctor looked at me with kind and sincere eyes, then said, "I'm sorry."

"So what now? I just do chemotherapy, and it goes away?" I asked, almost begging her to say *yes, chemotherapy would make it all go away.*

She took a deep breath before giving me my life sentence. "As of right now, this isn't curable, but it is treatable. You will have to live with this for the rest of your life."

I could tell this was just as hard for her to tell me as it was for my family and me to hear, but I just couldn't listen anymore. I sprinted out of the room, down the hallways, through the hospital doors, and collapsed to my knees in the grass at the edge of a beautiful garden.

Gasping for air, I cried, *Why, God! Why is this happening? Why now? I'm so young, and my life is just supposed to be starting.* My world as I knew it just came crashing down. *I am going to die. I don't want to. I still have so much life to live. I am not strong enough to go through this. I don't have it in me. If I have to die, it might as well just happen now. I don't want to graduate. I don't want to go to college. I just want this all to be over.*

Just as my spiraling thoughts started getting worse and worse, I saw Ben making his way over to me. He grabbed me and hugged me tight. I crumpled into his arms, my body shaking with sobs.

"I think you should break up with me." I started to say as I choked on my own tears.

He looked at me without a tear in his eye and said, "No. I am going to be here every step of the way. I know you are going to get through this. You are so much stronger than you realize, okay?"

It made me feel much better that he wasn't crying. When I was first diagnosed, he cried more than I did, so strangely, it made me more confident.

I stayed in the yellow and pink flower-filled garden for a while until my mom asked if I was ready to come back in. The doctor had something to tell me, so I mustered up the courage and walked back in there.

"Brittney, I know this is a scary diagnosis, but I have patients who are alive and well with this same disease since the 90s. There are more and more treatments coming out every day. The future is bright."

Her words spoke hope right into my heart and soul. *I am going to be one of those women.*

On the car ride home, my mom filled me in on everything the doctor said. The cancer was in my bones and liver. I had spots on my ribs, spine, pelvis, and sternum. I am ER-estrogen and HER2-positive. I am not sure what this means—it's all gibberish to me—but my mom explained this is what drives the cancer to grow.

I would have to undergo strong chemotherapy. Yes, it's official; I would lose my hair. After I finished chemo, I would remain on targeted treatment. I'd have an infusion once every twenty-one days for the rest of my life in hopes of keeping the cancer at bay. My doctor also wanted to start me on a hormone-blocking pill once a day—immediately.

I was really scared, but at the same time, I knew I'd be okay. I didn't know how to explain it, but I knew I would get through this. I had to. I had so much more to experience in life, and I had a world to help change.

Dear God,

Please help me through this.
I believe in you.
I believe in myself.
Please heal me from this disease.
Thank you in advance.
Love,

Brittney

Graduation Day

It's the morning of my first chemo session.
I notice the sunflowers on the wall by my infusion chair.
A sign of good luck?
Gratitude flows through my veins.
I smile and tell the nurse I am ready.
Also my name and date of birth.
Drip drip drip.
Lips go numb; I can't breathe.
Nausea takes over my stomach.
Mom races for the nurse.
Time for a little break and premeds.

All drugged up now.
Dizzy and tired,
Chemo starts again.
Time ticks by.
BEEP BEEP BEEP
Must be done for the day.
Just enough time to get ready for graduation.

White dress under my red cap and gown.
Everyone hugs me.
Congratulates me, but
One neighbor comes over and says,
My friend had MBC
Traveled to her brain
Then killed her
Good luck tonight, sweetie
Then leaves.

Happy and excited standing on the stage,
Surrounded by the peers I have grown with.
Speeches start to go on.
Our time and future are here, they all say.
Traveled to her brain
Still smiling but holding back tears,
I am happy for all my friends.
Their future is here.
But mine?
And then killed her
I don't know if I have one.

Present Moment

June 20th 2015

Life. Beautiful, bright, magical.

Today I am in the big apple with my mom,
niece, and grandpa for a day trip.
It's as if I am awake for the first time. I notice
everything that surrounds me.
The way the sun shines through the tree branches.
How the breeze feels as it makes my hair dance behind me.

I had the chance to visit the Statue of Liberty earlier today.
Now I sit on a park bench listening to the birds
sing their songs and watching people live.
A young boy skateboards back and forth in front of me,
a family of three lies in the grass under a tall tree, and
teenage girls try to get the perfect Instagram photo.

Seeing these people enjoy their lives expands
my heart with so much love.
I feel it in my chest, bursting.
I don't think I have ever seen the world
like this or even felt this way.
It's as if I'm *feeling* life.

This must be what it means to be fully present.

Thank you for this moment.

Magic of the Universe

The universe has always amazed me. I believe it draws the people you were supposed to meet into your life.

Whenever fear started to creep into my mind telling me that I would soon cease to exist, someone appeared out of nowhere with the hope I desperately needed.

A few days after graduation, my family and I left for a road trip to Florida. During the entire ride, I couldn't help but think about how I might not get to experience everything this life has to offer me. *What will the world be like without me? How will my family handle it?* So many haunting thoughts even though I was surrounded by the people I loved most and on my way to my favorite place.

On our way to Orlando, we always stopped at Daytona Beach, arriving just in time to see the sunrise. This time was no different. Once we got to the beach, my father parked. I jumped out of the van, grabbed my two-year-old niece, Rosie, and my boyfriend, Ben, and raced to the water.

My soul jumped up and down with excitement at the first step on the golden sand. When I reached the salty water, it became very still. Peace. At last. My family and I walked along the warm water as the sky began turning beautiful shades of pink and orange, reminding me of the everyday miracles in life.

With the sun now bright in the sky, Rosie walked over to a stranger and called him Papa. This was strange because that is what she calls my dad, who was in the van taking a nap. My mom ran over to apologize, but the man laughed and said it was okay because his children—also on the beach—called him that.

As we talked to the family more, my mom mentioned my story and how I was just diagnosed with metastatic breast cancer. To our surprise, the man and his family were very spiritual and called themselves "prayer warriors."

He gathered his entire family and mine right there on the beach. We formed a circle, all holding hands, and prayed together for my healing. It was beautiful, and at that moment, all my fear melted away. Love and gratitude flowed through my body for the rest of the trip, with the knowingness that I was okay.

Together

Today I woke up with my hair all over my pillow
Already?
One shower and it filled the drain
Only two weeks have passed since my first treatment
I cried
Ran a comb through my hair
Leaving strands tangled in the teeth
My heart sinks
For a moment of the day, I forget
I push my hair out of my face
Now it is in my fingers
I take a deep breath
And find my mom to shave it
She shaves hers with me
I am not alone
It is freeing
It is funny
And it is sad
All at once
But we did it together
Not alone

Dating Doctors

When you start dating, you realize not everyone is a good match for you. The same goes for doctors. You have to find one that feels right. It's basically dating.

I learned this the hard way when I met my first oncologist. She was distant and unresponsive, and when her PA made a mistake with my treatment, she yelled at my mom and me instead of taking responsibility. I saw the red flags waving in my face. I listened to my gut and found a new oncologist, one who truly cared about my well-being.

It was a hard decision, but I knew it was the right one.

On the way to his office, I passed a sign that said "Mountain of God." A reminder that I was in good hands. My mom had even reached out to a healer who told her to take me to the mountains, and here we were, the Mountain of God. The universe was sending me all the right signs.

But the real difference was in my doctor's approach. He *listened* to me, asked how I felt, and adjusted my treatment plan as needed. He even supported some of my complementary ways of healing— cannabis, herbs, diet, and so on. As long as what I was doing didn't affect my treatment in any way, he didn't see a problem with it. He treated me like a partner in my own care, not just a patient.

But my favorite thing about him was his *faith* in me.

When I asked him what stage my cancer was in, before answering, he looked me in the eyes and said, "Just remember, this is only a number." With compassion informed me I was considered stage 4. He also reminded me that I might encounter bumps on the road along the way, but we would get over them together.

I swear I left every appointment feeling a little lighter.

I was blessed by my medical team, especially my oncologist. Good doctors are out there; you may just need to meet some frogs first.

Inner Peace

Dr. S, my new oncologist, set me up with an appointment to speak to an oncologist in Boston because he wanted to ensure I received the best treatment for my cancer at my age. His doing that made me feel safe and confident that I would receive the best care possible. My healing was number one, not his pride or something he read in a textbook many years ago.

My mom and I were so excited to go to Massachusetts. We took my 2014 Silver Kia Soul and spent the day in Salem before I had my appointment the next day.

I love Salem. It's everything spooky and witchy. So, of course, we had to check out the Witch House and do some cool tours while there.

We stayed in a charming hotel that resembled a dollhouse, which we absolutely loved.

The following day, we drove to Boston for my appointment. I wasn't sure what to expect from the doctor, but it turned out to be quite different from what I had anticipated.

When I arrived, I checked in and sat in the waiting room with my mom until my name was called. When I heard my name, we both sat up and followed the young woman into a room. There she took my blood pressure, got my weight, and asked me a few questions before she left the room.

My mom and I didn't have to wait long before we heard the knock on the door.

My stomach did a little flip, so I inhaled and reminded myself I could do this. I hated going over my diagnosis, and in the last few months, that's all I ever did. Doctor after doctor, nurse after nurse, even family members, but I prepared myself for this one, and we even went to Salem first so that it wouldn't feel like a serious medical trip.

When he walked in, he shook my hand, introduced himself to us, and of course, mentioned how baffling it was that I had breast cancer at such a young age.

"Are you ready to get into this, Brittney? There are some serious things we need to talk about." He said while darting his eyes from me to my mom.

"Yeah, let's do it," I said, shooting him my famous finger guns.

"Yeah," my mom mustered. Even though I knew she wasn't ready to do this dance again.

We started talking about how serious this diagnosis is, treatment options, how there's no cure, but it's treatable, everything I already heard.

There was still one topic I never asked about—fertility. I figured now was the best time to ask.

"I have a question."

He looked at me and gave me a nod to go ahead and ask it.

"I am still holding on to hope for having kids one day. How will my chemo treatment and any future treatments I may need affect my fertility? Should I consider preserving my eggs?"

"Well, you know, statistically speaking, with this disease, you only have about three years to live, so who would take care of your children when you are gone?"

Feeling a bit taken aback by the comment just made, I looked him right into his eyes and said, "I am not going anywhere. I know what the statistics say, but I am a real person, and I know I will be here for a long time."

He looked at me with surprise and responded, "Well, we can only hope."

I kindly smiled at him and confidently responded, "No, I know I will be."

"We can try, but statistically, that is not likely."

I flashed him my beautiful smile with a side of chuckle and said, "I will be, and I understand that you can never feel the faith I have inside me, that's my feeling from God, and that you are a doctor who must go by the statistics, but thank you for your time."

And at that moment, I knew how strong I was and how my inner peace was unshakable. I felt my faith growing even stronger inside of me. And I felt no anger towards him.

When the appointment was over, Mom and I got in the car. I looked at her and started busting out laughing. "Well, that went well," I said sarcastically. "I can't believe he said that when I just wanted to know about fertility."

"Yeah, what was that?" My mom said with a hurt look. "Don't listen to him."

"Oh, I'm not. I am actually completely fine. It didn't affect me at all."

On the car ride home, I felt something expanding within me, like a ball of light encompassing me. It was a feeling of knowing I was going to be okay and that I shouldn't worry. The only way to describe it was pure LOVE.

Energy Healing

My friend Jen was nothing shy of a miracle worker. I started attending her meditation and law of attraction workshops when I was fifteen. Every single Sunday, I sat my little butt on a meditation pillow in her shop, Balance. Without even knowing, she helped me heal from my eating disorder, depression, and even helped me discover my own path into energy work.

At the beginning of my cancer diagnosis, I stopped going to meditation because I was so busy showing up for all my doctor appointments I forgot to show up to my *soul* appointments.

One Sunday, she texted me to check in because she noticed I hadn't been there in a while. I explained my current reality, and she told me if I showed up that night, it would be special. Filled with curiosity, I went and brought along Ben and my mom. If it was going to be special, I wanted them there too.

I walked into the candle-lit room and saw about fifteen people sitting on the floor with their backs against the wall, ready to meditate. I gave Jen a giant hug and then took my spot on the floor. She read a passage from *A Course in Miracles* and then guided us through a beautiful healing meditation.

"Start to wiggle your fingers and toes, maybe turning your head left to right. Take one more deep breath in, and when you are ready, you may open your eyes," Jen said soothingly to bring us back into the room.

I always felt a little disoriented after meditating but in the best way possible. I sometimes go so deep it feels weird when I return back to this world.

I opened my eyes and saw Jen looking at me with a huge smile. "My beautiful Brittney here is healing from breast cancer, and I wanted to do something special for her tonight. If you feel called to, I invite you all to stay for a healing circle."

My right hand instantly flung over my heart space as I felt it start opening. *Of course, Jen would surprise me with a healing circle. That was love. That was what we humans do for each other, and I couldn't think of something more beautiful than that.*

Everyone stayed, gathered in a circle, holding hands. I was in the middle as they all sent me healing energy. Holding me in their mind as whole and already healed. The energy sent didn't just go to the person in the middle; it flowed into everyone who participated in the circle. I felt light, as if every atom in my body was vibrating. The love was strong and pure.

Jen started offering healing circles more often. Sometimes I didn't even go into the middle because I didn't think I needed the extra healing—I knew in my heart I was already healed. With her help, I started healing from the inside out, the mind, body, and soul.

Mission Light

As strange as it is, I am so damn happy.
Everyone expects me to be curled up in a ball
in a dark room somewhere, but instead,
I'm running in a field of flowers and laughing with joy.

When you get sick, you appreciate everything so much more.
The cup of coffee in the morning,
Your superhero mother,
The air that fills your lungs.

Every morning you wake is miraculous.

I wish I could share this feeling I have with every single person.
I bet there would be a lot less illness,
violence, and suicides in this world.

Maybe this is my mission.

Maybe this illness came to open my eyes.
So I see this world for what it truly is,
then share the light I feel inside.

New Found Love

Bald and boobless never looked and felt so good. I updated my wardrobe and bought so many cute little flowy skirts, tops, dresses, and head scarves to wear. I felt confident with my pale bald head out for all to see, but sometimes a little scarf pulls the outfit together. Who would have thought cancer would be the thing to help me see the beauty I have shining inside?

A few months ago, I had a perfect fit body, with double D's and long shiny hair, but I was sad.

Looking in the mirror was hard. I hated the reflection I saw every day. So I starved myself and used makeup to hide.

I once thought being skinny, pretty, and having lots of friends would make me happy, but in reality, that wasn't true. Throughout my life, I felt empty—as if a part of me was missing—and I tried to fill it with the approval of others. Surely if others thought I was enough, I would too. But at the end of the day, I still felt worthless.

Losing all the parts I thought made me who I was, was freeing. I felt light for the first time in years and no longer cared what others thought because I realized it just didn't matter. I do not need the approval of anyone other than myself.

I looked in the mirror and saw a girl who was almost unrecognizable. The long brown hair was replaced with peach fuzz. The large chest was flat and covered with scars. My toned body, which I once worked so hard for, was now a bit softer.

But the biggest difference I saw in the mirror was the newfound confidence, happiness, and *love* that shone through me. I was no longer the unsure, sad girl who hated who she was.

I wouldn't trade this for the world.

The Day I Was a Tomato

Today, I had my fourth treatment and another bad reaction.

I was sitting in my little chair reading *Conversations with God* by Neale Donald Walsch when I suddenly couldn't breathe. My lips went tingly, my stomach queasy, and my face felt like someone lit it on fire. Panicked, I looked at my mom, who was on the phone with my nonna. As soon as she saw me, she dropped the phone and ran for the nurse. They stopped treatment immediately and put me on oxygen. My mom told me my face and chest looked like a tomato.

I can't imagine how hard it was for my mom to watch poison coursing through my veins. I knew I would be okay, but I also knew it was harder for my mom because she didn't share that inner gut feeling that I had. I wished I could place my hand on her heart and transfer my sense of knowingness and peace to her so she could have the same level of trust in my healing that I had.

I continued with the oxygen for ten minutes. Dr. S. came to talk to me, and thirty minutes later, I started treatment again with a slower drip. They also loaded me up with Benadryl, which knocked me out for the remainder of the treatment. Not going to lie; I kinda liked those naps.

The Bad Days

It's day two post-treatment, and I feel
lifeless, just a shell of a human.
My body feels like 1,000 pounds.
No matter how much I try to sleep, I never feel rested.
These are the days I don't feel like myself.

As I lie in bed, I feel a pang of jealousy.
I see my friends enjoying their summer,
Soaking up the sun at the beach,
Dancing the night away at concerts.

Meanwhile, I am trapped in bed.
Cancer roams my body, and chemo floods my veins.

I want so badly to wake up,
For this to be only an awful nightmare.

I just want to be healthy.

Tornado

Sometimes I know exactly who I am.
I feel unlimited, magical, and inspired.
Then out of nowhere, something inside switches,
and I no longer know who I am.

I am scared and confused.
My mind is a tornado wrecking everything in its path.
I have lost my sense of peace.
I can't sleep, and I am left with nothing
but thoughts of self-pity.

Reiki

I started having weekly reiki sessions with Jen, and they were magical.

Reiki is a form of energy healing that uses the practitioner as a tube for the energy to flow from Source—the Universe, God, or whatever name works for you. The energy flows through the practitioner's palms to the patient with either a hands-on, touching the body, or hands-off, not touching the body, technique. Most of the time, people feel the heat from the energy moving through the body and may even see certain colors, visions, or emotions. Or a person may feel nothing but relaxation. No matter what the experience, it works the same.

When I first arrived, Jen sat me down on her big comfy couch and asked me how I was feeling. Honestly, I was feeling rundown, and those pesky "what if" thoughts were starting to creep up on me, drowning me in the world of cancer. Every thought and feeling, both physically and mentally, were about cancer, and I couldn't escape. I was getting pulled under.

I explained it all to her, and she told me to be gentle with myself. She said feelings come and go like waves on the beach, and we would work on letting them go. She took me back to her reiki room, and I slipped off my shoes and climbed onto the black massage table. I covered myself with a thin tie-dyed blanket, took a few deep breaths, and closed my eyes. She ran her pendulum over all seven of my energy centers and told me I was off balance, but by the time we were done, I would be flowing like a rockless river.

During the treatment, her hands radiated heat in each spot she touched as if she had lit a match. I saw a beautiful white healing light enter and swirl through my body, and I allowed anything that no longer served me to flow out.

After the treatment, I slowly opened my eyes and sat up, feeling as light as a feather. I'm not sure if it was the treatment itself that made me feel that way or just being in Jen's presence. She carried a certain energy that just felt good. She's one powerful soul, and I'm very thankful for her sharing her light with me.

Friends Who Are There

Bliss. Pure Bliss.
In a car full of my best friends
Blasting Biggie Smalls
Thirty miles an hour
Eyes closed
Arms opened wide
Wind hitting my bald head
Standing out of Paige's sunroof
Mind clear
This moment is Bliss
Pure Bliss.

Peace

Peace is my goal.
The kind of inner peace that not even
my darkest hour can shake.
The kind that even on the outside, when things
seem like chaos and nothing is going right,
I still believe in possibility.
Possibility so great that only the Universe can conspire,
but I still trust in it.
Trust that everything is going to work out for my greatest good,
as long as I keep hanging in there,
as long as I keep going,
as long as I can find even the smallest
thing to hold gratitude for.
Peace is what I seek.

Feel

I used to push away any fear, sadness, or anger,
because I thought feeling it made me weak,
but now I realize it is part of the healing process.

It's okay to feel.
To be sad or angry.
In fact, we must allow ourselves
to move through all arising emotions.
Putting on a fake smile and pretending
to be happy does nothing.

So I say ...

Let the tears fall.
Punch the pillow.
Let it all out.
And when you're ready ...
Release it.

Feel the feelings, but don't become them.

The Seeds Were Left

Like the lotus flower, a natural disaster came and wiped me out. I thought my life was over, and so did whoever looked at me. I appeared to have lost my roots from the flood of cancer mixed with a cocktail of chemo. Bald, no eyelashes or eyebrows, dark rings around my eyes, no breasts, and tired beyond belief, nothing seemed left of me. But there was—when the cancer receded and only my soul was left—the seed of my body was still there. A piece of me died, but I was being reborn into something much better and happier.

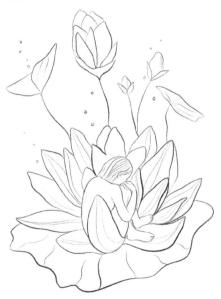

Pink Out

"There is no evidence of disease! You can stop now!"

Those were the most beautiful words I'd ever heard.

I was at my high school's "pink out" football game. Everyone wore pink, including the football players and the cheerleaders. Money was raised to help someone in the community undergoing breast cancer treatment. We had this game every year, but this year was extra special.

I was excited to attend not only to help the cause but also to see some friends I went to high school with. I stood by the cheerleaders celebrating a touchdown scored by the boys in red and blue—the Vikings—and then I felt my phone vibrate. I looked down and saw it was a New York number. It was already 10 pm, so I almost didn't answer, but something told me I should.

"Hello?"

"Hi, Brittney. This is Dr. Wang."

"Oh, Hi! Is everything okay?" I asked immediately. I felt my stomach starting to knot up.

"I know it's late, but I just got a look at your scan results."

My heart sank. I felt my palms getting sweaty. "Oh, how does it look?" I asked hesitantly, unsure if I wanted to know the answer.

"I am amazed by them. It showed there is no evidence of disease! You can stop Taxotere now!"

Even with a crowd of people around me, tears started to fill my eyes.

"Oh, my God!! Thank you for taking time out of your night to tell me this."

"I already spoke to Dr. S. about this. We are both very happy and agree your next treatment will be the very last one with Taxotere. After that, we will continue you on the other treatments, H and P, every three weeks, along with your daily pill. If you need anything at all, give me a call. I will continue to monitor you." Then Dr. Wang said goodbye and hung up.

When I got off the phone, everyone around me asked if I was okay. I waved my arms in the air and screamed with excitement, "I have no evidence of disease in my body!"

Everyone around me started congratulating me with tight hugs.

Growing Through Mud

I was born anew, but the healing process from all the trauma
I just experienced wasn't easy. Like the lotus flower, I had
to grow through mud before the sun could shine on me.

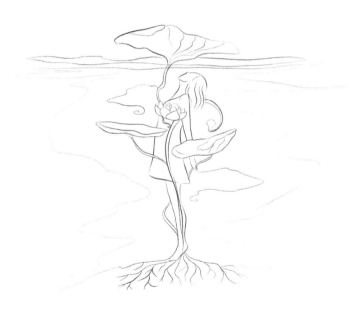

Scared and Confused

Despite receiving the incredible news that my body no longer showed evidence of active disease and that I could stop Taxotere, I couldn't shake off the feeling of terror that washed over me. It wasn't that I didn't feel joy—I was over the moon—but when the excitement settled down, I realized I was terrified at the same time.

I wonder if I should do a few more rounds of chemo just to be sure nothing is left to decrease my chances of progression.

My mind was all over the place. I wasn't even sure if extra dosing as a precaution was a thing.

When I mentioned how I was feeling to Ben, he got angry. "You are the healthiest you are ever going to be! There is no reason for you to be sad."

Those words cut like a sharp knife. I was already confused by my feelings, but now I felt like my emotions were invalid. They are wrong and shouldn't be felt. Was something wrong with me? Would anyone else just simply feel joy?

That would be nice. Tie cancer up with a neat little bow and be done with it, but that's not the reality. Even if I wasn't stage 4, it's not that simple.

The thing is, what he said hit the nail on the head. I was the healthiest I would ever be, and that sent shivers down my spine. It could only go downhill from here. What if the second I stopped this treatment, the cancer woke up and started growing?

I was scared.

10-21-15

"Last Day Of Taxotere!"
Mom created this sign in bright pink bubble letters.
It is difficult, but I choose to release fearful
thoughts and replace them with new ones.

What if I stop treatment and live a happy and healthy life?

What would that look like?

I would—no, I AM—opening a retreat
center for people just like me.
People experiencing a tough time in life, mentally or physically.
I will be there to hold their hand.

I am helping to change the world for the better.
I am traveling the entire world, learning
about beautiful cultures.
I am writing a book.
I am moving to Florida and living on a beach.
I am getting married and having beautiful babies.
I am living.

I create my own reality.

Creating Happiness

I was lounging on the couch, wrapped up in my wool blanket, lost in thoughts about what to do with my life now that I had finished my last chemo session. I wasn't in school or working and felt a bit lost. As if by fate, a Universal Studios commercial popped up on my TV, and it struck me—I knew where I wanted to go.

I threw off my blanket, jumped off the couch, and rushed to tell my mom, who was teaching her kindergarten class in the kitchen. Just as I started to open my mouth, she gave me a finger-to-lips warning to be quiet. I gave her a thumbs-up to indicate that I had a great idea brewing.

With out-of-control butterflies in my stomach, I saw myself lying in the warm sun by the beautiful palm trees while waiting for her class to end.

"Hey, Britt! What do you want? My class is over," Mom asked as she entered the living room.

"Okay, hear me out! I just saw a Universal Studios commercial and think we are overdue for a Florida trip! It is cold here, and we haven't celebrated my last Taxotere treatment yet!" I tried my best to convince her.

She smiled, let out a little chuckle, and said, "I agree! I saw the same commercial yesterday and started looking up hotels! I actually found a nice condo available, but it's for this upcoming week."

I exploded with excitement! "Let's go! You ask Dad, and I'll ask Ben! It will be so much fun!"

Her face lit up. "Okay, let's do it!"

Just like that, we had a *just do it* moment. Ben and I worked at Wendy's, and the manager understood my situation. He allowed Ben to have the week off with only two days' notice. My dad is his own boss, so he had no trouble getting time off.

Cancer taught me to live life in the present and pursue what truly made me happy. I hope to keep doing that for the rest of my days.

Learning Patience

Walking around Disney and Universal used to be a breeze for me from the moment they opened until the last firework, but that wasn't the case anymore.

When I finished my last Taxotere treatment, I thought things would return to normal. I thought my energy levels would instantly rise and my hair would grow back as fast and long as ever. But that didn't happen. In fact, my eyelashes and eyebrows fell out after my last treatment. It felt like a setback.

Leaving Universal Studios, I felt defeated. We didn't even stay until close, and I was exhausted. The walk back to the car felt like an eternity. Every step I took felt like I had bricks weighing me down. I tried not to show it, but I was disappointed in myself for not lasting the entire day.

I think Ben realized I was upset because he looked at me with the most sincere eyes and said. "You have no hair, no eyebrows, no makeup, and are dripping in sweat, but you are still the most beautiful girl I have ever seen."

He always knew exactly what to say to light me up inside. I hugged him, closing my eyes and embracing all the love he had to give me. I took a deep breath, looked him in the eyes, and thanked him. That was what I needed—to remember to be kind to myself.

It had been challenging since I stopped chemo and was now "no evidence of disease" (NED). Where did this leave me? I was the healthiest I will ever be, but I was still on targeted treatments and still had lasting effects from chemo.

I didn't have all the answers, but I knew the best thing I could do was take it day by day and relearn how to live life. I would never be the same and needed patience while becoming the new me. This would be my forever journey, and I needed to learn to accept the things I could not change.

Another Year of Life

December 5th 2015

"Haapppyyyy birthdaaay tooo youuu," my mom sang
as she entered my room with shiny birthday balloons,
waking me up for the day with excitement.

I'm nineteen today! Another day lived. Another *year* of *life*.

I used to be scared of getting older, but now
I understand what a blessing it is.

I want all the birthdays and years—even the
wrinkles and gray hairs they bring.

Give me them all, baby!

Maybe not the wrinkles and gray hair just *yet*,

but one day, I will welcome them.

I roll out of bed.
My feet hit the floor.
Gratitude shook my body.
Thank you.
Thank you.
Thank you.

I set an intention as I brush my teeth.

Today, I will be present and cherish each moment.

For this year ahead, I want to live my life.

I will take risks and be who I am unapologetically.
I want to travel and love with all my heart.
I want to experience everything.
My intention is to *feel* life every day.

I spend the day with my family, eating fluffy birthday pancakes and shopping.

Mom surprised me with a party.
Seeing all my friends and family together in one place made my heart flutter.

A big rectangular cake with white frosting, rainbow sprinkles, "Happy birthday, Brittney," glittered in pink icing.

Everyone gathers around to sing to me
I smile like a giddy child.

I blow out my candles
wishing for another year of good health.

Happy 19th year of life to me.

To Let Go or Keep Trying

You know when you can feel someone slipping away from you, and it hurts so deep it hurts your insides? I felt Ben slowly disappearing from my life. The pain of losing him crept up on me, gnawing away at my insides. Two weeks passed since we saw each other, and every time I tried to make plans, he was too busy with his friends.

When we went out to eat a few weeks ago, I told him I was trying out a plant-based diet. He made a comment about how I was boring because I didn't eat "fun" food anymore. It may have been a small thing, but it hurt my feelings deeply. My world had been caving in on me the last few months, and I needed his support to lift it.

Then he told me he didn't know how he felt about me anymore. He said I changed and admitted I was a better person now but no longer necessarily the person for him. I tried to get back to the girl I used to be for him, but I couldn't. I wasn't her anymore, and I don't think I wanted to be.

A Leap of Faith

Ever since I was little, I wanted to go skydiving. Growing up, my mom and I talked about it all the time. She said once I turned eighteen, we would finally make the jump. Unfortunately, cancer stole that away from me as I was too sick to jump out of planes.

Now a year later, two months out of treatment, it was worth the wait.

Mom and I arrived in Florida the other day for a birthday getaway trip. I did not know she was planning for us to skydive!

She woke me up with my favorite breakfast—pancakes in the shape of Mickey—and told me the day had finally come, the day we skydived together.

I jumped out of bed with excitement, gave her a hug, and hurried to get ready. I threw on a pair of pink shorts and a pink shirt that said "Walking Miracle," and we were on our way to our biggest adventure yet.

The place was about an hour away, and I had butterflies doing loops in my stomach the entire drive. I thanked my mom repeatedly, letting her know this was the best surprise I had ever had. When we finally arrived, we filled out waivers and sat through a safety video with our instructors. My instructor was a tall skinny man built like Gumby with long blonde hair and a beard. His name was Bob. My mom had a short, younger man, Craig, with piercing blue eyes. Just as we put on the harnesses and strapped to our instructors, we learned it was too cloudy, and we had to wait for the sky to clear up.

I was crushed. We were so close, and now we might not get to do it. Once again, something totally out of my control blocked me from living out this dream. An hour passed, and it was not looking good. I was growing restless and about to call it a day and go back to the hotel, but my mom convinced me to wait a little bit longer. She still had faith it would clear up.

Sitting at a wooden picnic table, I closed my eyes and took a few deep breaths. I asked the Universe if I was meant to do this today, to help the clouds clear up and reveal the beautiful sun that was hiding behind them. I felt gratitude in my heart and let the Universe do its thing, releasing my attachment to the outcome.

Within the next half an hour, the instructors walked up to us and told us it was time! The butterflies were now back, fluttering intensely. Mom looked at me and asked, "You ready?"

I nodded my head and started to put my harness back on. Then I started to question my sanity as we walked towards the plane.

Oh God, Oh God. What am I doing? Am I crazy?

The second I stepped foot on the plane, my mind went quiet, and gratitude once again took over. *Finally,* I thought. My mom, on the other hand, looked terrified. Two other people loaded the plane with us, another mother and her daughter duo. We straddled the wide seat, and the instructors began attaching themselves to us.

When the plane started going, I realized we were going backward and blurted out, "Oh my gosh, is the plane flying backward?"

Bob laughed and said, "We are sitting backward," then turned around to point to the pilot.

"Oh, it must be my nerves," I said, feeling embarrassed.

He then told me I was in charge of opening the parachute.

I looked at him like he was crazy, chuckled, and said, "Do you want to die? I will kill us."

"No, you won't. I will let you know when to pull it."

As we started to get higher and higher, all I could say was, "Wow. This is truly amazing." Twenty minutes later, we reached 13,500 feet. It was time. My mom jumped first, and then it was my turn.

I put on my safety goggles, and my instructor and I scooted to the door. He asked me if I was ready and told me on three, we would jump. One—I took a deep breath in. Two—released the breath through my mouth. Three—smiling from ear to ear, we dove into the clear blue sky.

I expected my stomach to drop, but it didn't. It was exhilarating! I felt free as the cold wind hit my face. The smell of the air was fresh and crisp, and the view, my God, the view was breathtaking. Falling through the sky, seeing the white fluffy clouds around us and the fields of green grass and lakes below us was surreal. This is what I have been waiting my whole life to do.

I opened my arms wide and surrendered to the sky, trying to take it all in. In what seemed like only seconds but was 5,000 feet later, Bob tapped me on the shoulder, letting me know to pull the parachute. I slightly panicked but quickly regained control and pulled the strap for the parachute to open.

It felt like the sky pulled us back up, but it was just the canopy slowing us down. I noticed the clouds and realized they looked like the stuffing in a teddy bear. Bob tried to guide us through a cloud, but it didn't work, so he showed me some cool tricks in the sky. One was called "rollercoaster," and even let me help steer the parachute.

After about four minutes of falling slowly through the sky, it was time to land. Bob told me to position my body as if I were sitting on a chair and then lift my legs as high as I could. I did as I was told, and Bob took over the rest. As we neared the ground, I saw my mom waiting for me! I couldn't help but smile, and all of a sudden, I felt a thud. We landed safely!

What an experience!
What a thrill!
What a life!

I ran to my mom, hugged her, and told her I would do it all over again. She agreed she would too.

I felt like this jump represented me taking back my life. Taking back what I thought cancer stole. I finally felt like I had won.

Not because I have no evidence of disease, but because I was still choosing to live my life!

Flickering Light

Little by little, I see the signs, like a flickering
light threatening to go out.
I see the change in how you look at me,
the excuses not to see me that come too easily,
the silence that lingers between us.

I try to ignore what I see.
I believe the light can grow strong again because
out of the blue, you do a 180 and light me up with love again.

But this time is different.

You say you don't know how you feel,
that we need a break.

Then hours later, you call back,
asking to come over as if nothing had happened.

You are a broken switch damaging my light.

Now, I'm left in the dark,
uncertain of where we stand.
You say you love me,
but your actions speak louder than words.

I forgave you once, but the damage has been done.
The light that shined brightly between us is snuffed out,
replaced by emptiness and fear that makes my stomach churn.

January 4th

I lay in bed the night before my first PET
scan since being declared NED.
I feel nervousness and gratitude.
It felt like just yesterday I received the incredible news,
but now it's time to face the possibility of bad news once again.

It's like studying hard for a test and receiving an excellent score.
Relief at seeing the grade, but school
continues, and you learn a new topic.
This topic is harder than the last—you have less
help and support than you did before.
The pressure increases.
You got a good grade on the last test, but who
is to say you won't fail the next one?
Cancer is a never-ending school year;
you're in it for the rest of your life.

January 5th

And just like that, I aced another exam.
I am NED!!
No evidence of disease in this perfectly
healed, strong, beautiful body of mine.
Thank you.

Decisions

After doing extensive research on surgeons, I finally met with the winner, who will start reconstructing my chest. I had been flat for almost a year, and while I didn't mind it, I was finally ready to have this surgery.

To be honest, I was not sure if I wanted reconstruction for a few reasons. Most of the reasons were based on fears.

Reason 1- What if having this surgery triggers something and causes a recurrence?
Reason 2- What if something goes wrong in surgery?
Reason 3- What if my surgeon completely botches my chest?
Reason 4- Am I willing to gamble the self-love I've finally found for the first time?

I took these concerns with me when I met the surgeon. She helped answer my questions and gave me some relief.

1- She explained that the surgery itself wouldn't trigger a recurrence, but as any surgery does, it could lower my immune system. *Interesting. Something to think about.*

2- Again, just like any other surgery, it came with risks which she went over with me. Risks include infection, problems with the incisions not healing properly, blood clots, problems with the implants themselves, and so on. *Something to also think about.*

3- She showed me other work she had done to see if I liked it. *I am glad she showed me because this helped me have more confidence in her.*

4- This one, I tackled myself. When I sat and thought about it, I realized that if I truly learned to love myself, nothing could take that away from me. Of course, sometimes it could be a little harder, but at the end of the day, I should always return to the state of love. This body is MINE! Any shape, size, or modification I chose deserved to be celebrated and loved.

We discussed many topics at the appointment, and I left feeling pretty confident. I didn't make a decision right away. I told her I would go home and sit down with all the information. She agreed that was the best thing to do.

After talking things over with my mom, who came to the appointment with me, I decided to move forward, and we made a date to put my expanders in on February 16th, 2016.

Watch out, world, I was going to have boobs again!

Late Night Thoughts

The darkness of night amplifies the noise in my head,
making it impossible to sleep.

My mind wanders to Ben.
He was supposed to accompany Dad and me
to New York City to have my surgery.

But now, he's not coming, and I feel abandoned and alone.

Am I making the right decision by going through with the surgery?
What if something goes wrong?
What if I never wake up?

The fear of the unknown is all-consuming.

Maybe if I text Ben and try to fix things,
he will come with me, and everything will be okay.
I know I shouldn't have to beg someone to be there for me,
but I feel desperate for comfort right now.

The silence on the other end of the phone is deafening
but eventually, he replies and agrees to come.

It feels pathetic that I had to convince him to come,
but I need something to go right in my life,
even if it is just pretend.

Reflections

Standing before the mirror, I fixate on my flat, scarred chest.
Turning and tilting my body, I examine every angle
as if trying to piece together a puzzle that has been taken apart.

I glide my finger across the scars,
remembering the journey that has led me to this moment.

I envision myself with new breasts.

How will they feel? What will they look like?
Will they feel heavy, like my double D's?

My expanders will be placed tomorrow,
so I still have time to decide on size.

I close my eyes, inhale deeply, exhale slowly.
I whisper *I got this,*
Willing my words to take root.

I meet my reflection's gaze with a smile
and trust my decision for reconstruction.

Under Construction

The night before the surgery, my dad drove us to my cousin's house right outside the city, making the morning less stressful. On the morning of surgery, I checked in, and after waiting with my dad and Ben, a nurse came and told me it was time. She walked me to the operating room.

My stomach dropped as I entered the room. It was sterile, and I'm not talking about cleanliness. The room had plain white walls with just operating equipment and a table in the center. It felt soulless and scary. How strange to know in a few minutes, I would be opened up, exposed. As I hopped up on the table and leaned back, I thought my heart would jump out of my chest. I looked up and saw huge bright lights above me.

"You ready?" she asked.

I nodded my head, and she placed a mask over my nose and mouth. I counted back from one hundred, and the next thing I knew, I was out.

When I woke up after my surgery, I kept going in and out of consciousness. It was hard to stay awake. I opened my eyes once and saw Ben with a distraught look. When he noticed I was awake, he raced to my side to tell me he loved me. I told him I loved him too and then dozed off again. *I understood now.* He was so scared of losing me that he started to push me away.

I stayed the night in the hospital. The expanders caused my chest to feel tight, but the pain was much less than my mastectomy. To be honest, I think my emotional pain was worse than the physical one.

I again looked like an octopus—drains stuck out of my sides. I had to strip them myself and mark down how much fluid I drained. I was stuck with them for about a week, then needed to drive back to NYC to hopefully get them removed.

I was officially Under Construction.

The Cancer Blues

The days following my surgery felt like being stuck in a time loop. I lounged on the same couch, watching the same show for days trying my best not to rip out my drains. Every second, I checked them to make sure they were fully intact, and every second they still were.

I had no shower in my future. I had little hair and felt an egg could fry on my scalp.

My wardrobe consisted of gray sweatpants and a pink surgical bra filled with gauze. *Sexy.*

I knew I should be kind to myself during this healing process, but it was hard.

The only thing that made me feel better was Rosie. My little ray of sunshine. She crawled up on the couch with me, grabbed my hand, and dozed off with me. I had been praying for another miracle, and she was most definitely it.

Freedom from the Octopus

Cancer is a mindfuck. One day I was falling apart; the next, I was leaping for joy. The day my octopus arms were removed, I was a dancer leaping across the stage of life. Let freedom ring!

My surgeon praised my healing progress and gave me the green light for my first fill. We scheduled it for the end of the month, which meant I was one step closer to having new foobs—fake boobs. It was surreal to think that in a few months, I'd have a new body. The past year offered a whirlwind of emotions, but I remained hopeful this was the start of a new chapter in my life.

Since my parents and I were already in the city, we decided to make the most of our trip and explore. The only problem was that everyone walking by me was dressed like they were ready to walk the runway in New York fashion week, while I wore sweatpants, an oversized jacket, and a beanie. Yikes!

I felt out of place and uncomfortable with how I looked. But at the same time, *who cares.* No, seriously, who cares? No one! If all those people silently judged me, that is on them. I will most likely never see them again. So instead of letting my insecurities control my life, I put my ego aside and basked in my freedom and the joy of being alive in this beautiful city.

First Fill Giggles

I heard the process of getting fills was uncomfortable and a little painful. So before my first fill, I decided to eat a little bit of an edible to dodge the pain. Sidenote, I never had an edible before.

Walking into my appointment, I figured I didn't eat enough of the cookie. Either that or edibles aren't what everyone made them out to be. My mom and my niece went with me to my appointment, but I didn't tell her what was in the cookie I ate. It was my little secret.

After I checked in and was escorted to a room, I changed into a hospital gown, and the three of us patiently waited for the nurse. Rosie was being silly, trying to make us laugh, and it worked. Well, at least it did for me. Uncontrollable laughter bubbled up from deep inside. Rosie is funny, but she is not that funny.

"Brittney, are you okay?" My mom asked.

"Yeah, Rosie is just so funny," I said, giggling away.

Mom gave me a weird look and started questioning me but was interrupted by a knock on the door. The nurse walked into the room and greeted us. That is when I realized what was happening.

Oh shit. I am really high.

The giggles suddenly turned into panic.

Just act normal, Brittney.

After a thorough examination, the nurse said everything looked great, and I was ready for my first fill.

Oh my God. She is totally going to know.

She first located the center of the expander and then used a black marker to mark the point of access. She grabbed one scary-looking needle with a giant syringe attached to it.

"Are you ready?" She asked.

I just smiled and nodded.

"Alright. Here we go." She began poking the needle into my right "breast," then slowly pushed saline into the expander.

"You doing okay?"

"Yeah, it isn't as bad as I thought it would be."

"Gooood," she said with a smile.

When she was done, she repeated the procedure on my left side, and then we were done.

My chest was numb, so I didn't feel anything but pressure. Also, I was high as a kite.

After grabbing a quick bite to eat, my mom, Rosie, and I took a taxi out of the city to my cousin's house, where our car was parked. I put on my headphones to listen to music for the hour ride there. Getting out of the taxi, I realized I never hit play on my music. I was listening to nothing the entire way. What a day.

How

The worst part of a breakup
is when the person who understood you best
becomes nothing but a stranger you once knew.

Just another memory.

Breakup

"Are we still hanging out today? We need to talk."

"We might later. I am eating Chinese food with the guys."

"Can you give me at least ten minutes to talk on the phone?"

"Yeah, later, though."

"Just so you know, you are hurting me more by ghosting me
rather than if you just broke up with me.
It hurts so much that you are dragging this out.
I can't do it anymore.
I think we should just end it now."

"Okay. It's not that I don't love you, though.
I just really don't know what I want to do with my life."

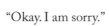

"You should have just told me you wanted to break up
instead of not talking to me for days.
It's whatever, though.
Shit happens.
People grow apart.
Maybe one day we will return to one another,
or maybe we won't.
Who knows.
Best of luck to you while you figure out your life.
Goodbye."

"Okay. I am sorry."

And that was it.

Calm Before the Storm

After ending things with Ben, I felt like a weight lifted off my shoulders. I woke up feeling empowered and confident, twirling around my house and singing "Love Myself" by Hailee Steinfeld at the top of my lungs. Every lyric leaving my body made the emotions in me grow stronger. I realized how much better I deserved than a confused love. I deserved the same love I gave. So until I received it from someone else, I'd give all my love to me.

I also noticed a new sense of self-confidence. I had cleavage, and I wasn't afraid of showing it off! I played Beyonce's "Feelin' Myself" on repeat and strutted around the house.

And to top it off, I decided to treat myself to some amazing experiences. I impulsively booked a ten-day trip to Italy in the summer and a week-long all-inclusive stay in Cancun with my mom for my birthday. What adventures might lie ahead? All I knew was that I was ready to take on the world and embrace all the love and joy it offered. Here's to new beginnings!

The One

Why do people think there's only one person for them?
Think of all the souls you can fall in love with.
The world is vast,
and you will go through many heartbreaks
before you find the one.
The one who won't leave you,
hurt you,
or break your beautiful heart.
You won't have to chase them or convince them to love you.
They will just stay and be right by your side
to take on life together.
Trust me.
The right love will be better than you have ever imagined.

The Broken Part

Damaged Goods.
Unlovable.
Broken.

I now live with an invaded body.
One that can be attacked at any time.
What do people do when war breaks out?
They flee.
They flee for their lives.
Just as Ben did.

He said he loved me so much,
But in the end,
It was easy for him to go.
To walk away like I meant nothing.

Leaving me feeling . . .
Abandoned.
Lonely.
Empty.

I am a burden to love.

Moving Backward

I healed from this self-hatred.
I beat it.
Remember?
I love myself now.

So, why am I sitting here hating myself
for every scar I see
and every negative thought running through my mind?
I am not supposed to think this way.
I am positive now.

But I didn't go to college.
I am gaining weight.
My hair is short, messy, and has no style.

Ben left me.
My own body tried to kill me.
I am not doing enough.
I am a loser.
I am failing at life.
I hate myself all over again.

But wait.

I healed from this.
Didn't I?

Going Forward

I read somewhere that when you go through
something traumatic or heal from depression, your
brain tries to suck you back into the sad emotions.

It's addicted to those feelings.
The feeling is familiar.

So when you start getting better, happiness
and peace are unknown to the brain.
The brain's not comfortable with it.
So it brings up old memories and emotions it knows you know.
You just keep repeating the same patterns over again.

It takes work to break yourself out of old feelings and responses
because, in the moment, you don't realize you're self-sabotaging.

Healing isn't always easy,
but it is worth it,
and it is possible.

I am not giving up on myself.
I will move forward even when I experience setbacks.
This is *my* life, and I deserve to be happy.

Masterpiece

I was broken and trying to pick up the pieces and force them back together again. I didn't realize they wouldn't fit together like they once did. They changed. I'm not the same person I once was, so why was I so desperately trying to make them fit?

It's hard sometimes to release old parts of you, but you must grow and evolve. Once you let go of those old pieces that no longer fit into the masterpiece you are, you can start creating new pieces that will flow so perfectly that you wonder why it was hard to let go in the first place.

You realize you were never broken, just changing.

California

My first time in California, I got off the plane and ran into someone who was Internet famous. I stared for a while until I finally found the courage to ask for a picture. I immediately got high hopes that I'd bump into Beyonce? A girl could dream.

On a real note, my trip to California had a purpose beyond celebrity sightings.

I was invited to a photo shoot for the Haus of Volta's Survivor Pinup Calendar. Every year they make a calendar that showcases breast cancer survivors and thrivers to help them reclaim their beauty and sensuality. The founder's story of her own journey of accepting her body after breast cancer resonated with me, and I was humbled to be asked to be a part of something that also helps raise awareness that young women can and do get breast cancer.

But of course, my trip couldn't be solely based around something with cancer, my mom came along, and we planned to explore Disneyland! Being a Disney fanatic, what else would you expect?

Pinup Babe

An itty bitty white bikini, stilettos, glam, and a hot pink car sum up my experience. Oh, and men honking at me in front of my mom as I attempted to be sexy.

It. Was. Amazing.

Minus the men.

Stori, the founder, glammed my face with makeup. I don't wear much, so as I sat in the chair watching her use product after product, my palms started to sweat. The thought *I am going to look like a clown* passed through my mind a few times. She must have felt my anxiety because, at one point, she looked at me and reassured me I was looking great.

When she was done, she turned my chair around for the final reveal in the mirror. I gasped when I saw the reflection looking back at me.

The first words out of my mouth were, "I look beautiful!" Followed by, "Thank you." I smiled as I checked myself out.

I was fully glammed. My eyebrows were perfect, my eyeshadow looked like art on my face, and I had a fake pair of long, full eyelashes and a beautiful shade of pink lipstick. I looked good.

Now it was time for my outfit. She gave me the tiniest little white bikini, yellow stilettos with a cute little blue bow on the toes, and big pink earrings. The confidence from a second ago disappeared. *No way I am going to look good in that.*

Before walking out to show everyone how I looked, I stared at myself in the mirror for a solid five minutes trying to raise the confidence to step out. I ran my fingers over my soft tummy, telling myself I should have worked out more.

"Brittney, are you okay?" my mom asked from the other side of the door.

"Yeah, I am coming out now!" I responded as I glanced once more in the mirror and stumbled out. "Here I am!" I said while doing a little spin to show a 360 view.

"You look amazing!" said Stori.

"Yeah, you do!" her daughter confirmed.

"The bikini fits you so well!" my mom assured me.

I smiled and thanked them as my confidence began to grow.

We walked outside, and in the grass was a hot pink convertible with a huge engine on the front.

For the first photo, I sat on the car's hood and smiled, not really knowing how to pose or what to do.

"Come on, move around, feel yourself!" The photographer encouraged me.

I realized I was showing how insecure I was, so in that moment, I decided to fake it to make it.

I crawled up on the car and started posing. *I am a model. I am beautiful.* I affirmed to myself pose after pose.

Before I knew it, I felt the words and radiated confidence. *My scars are sexy. I am breathtaking.*

"YES!" The photographer cheered. "Work it!"

At this point, men started honking at me. I hated it, but it wasn't going to get in my way of having fun. I continued to pose, knowing I looked good.

We deserve to feel good in our skin after cancer. Feminine and sexy, scars and all.

If we believe in our beauty, no one else can tell us otherwise.

When the shoot was done, I felt a sense of pride and gratitude. I proved to myself confidence comes from within. I participated in something bigger than myself, bigger than my insecurities. I hoped I could inspire other cancer thrivers to feel proud and confident in their own bodies.

Stori and her daughter are kind, genuine, and uniquely who they are. They reminded me I don't have to conform to anyone else's expectations. Each of us is perfect just as we are.

The Healing Part

Slowly I start to patch my broken heart.

I made it through times that stripped me bare,
when my heart was full of pain and sorrow,
and I wanted to give up on myself.

Skipped treatments that upset my mom,
Long self-loathing walks around Lake Scranton,
and every night, my hopes shattered anew
when the "I miss you" call or text never came.

All this leads me to where I am now.

I discover more about myself each day.
I know I am strong enough on my own.
I realize he is not a villain, and I am not a victim.
People sometimes grow apart.
I will forever be grateful for the time we shared,
But I'm finally okay without him.

It's one of the most painfully beautiful times in my life.

I Am My Superhero

This is the part where I find my power.
Where I fall in love with who I am.
Where I get comfortable with being on my own.
I am my superhero.

Tips for a Breakup

- Cry. Cry again. Cry some more. Don't hold back the tears. You need to let them fall.

- Feel. Let the emotions come up. The bad and the good. Holding them in is never a good idea because you'll never fully heal.

- Let your family and friends hold you up. Do not try to go through this alone. It is okay to ask for help. Breakups are difficult, and your loved ones want to be there for you. Often when we are in a relationship, we spend all of our time with our beloved, so it will feel really good to hang out with your friends again.

- Get comfortable with your own company. This is an amazing time to get to know yourself better. Who are you? Who do you want to be? Take up a new hobby or take yourself on a date. Fall in love with yourself.

- Do not stalk your ex. If it is a bad breakup, it might be best to delete this person's number and sever social media ties. It is not healthy to continually text long paragraphs on how you feel. Maybe once for closure, but then let it go. Do not look at their social media to check up on them. Just do not do it. At that point, you are just breaking your own heart over and over again.

- Accept it. It might have been the most amazing relationship you ever had, but for some reason, it just didn't work out, learn to be okay with it. I promise you'll find someone even better than you thought out there for you, even if you can't imagine it right now.

A Gift

Health is the greatest gift in life
Many take it for granted
Your heart beating in your chest
Your lungs expanding
Allowing you to take each breath
All the cells in your body working exactly as they were designed
You can take on anything
Do whatever your heart and soul desire
That is the ultimate gift
Health.

Swapped

Expanders out, bags of silicone in
Surgery went smoothly
I am bruised, swollen, and sore
But
I am also
Relieved, pleased, and thankful

Dance Party

You know those days when you think,
Wow, this is my life,
and throw a pity party for everything wrong?

Yeah, I almost did that.

But the second I started feeling sorry for myself,
I took a step back, zoomed out, and realized,
Wow! This is my life!
So much good surrounds me.

At that moment, my heart and soul filled with gratitude.

It's easy to throw a pity party,
but it feels better to throw a dance party.

Summer

This summer is the best of my life

Countless beach trips
Warm sand beneath my toes, sounds of waves crashing
Beautiful bright sun in the sky
Peace

Friends
Long nights laughing so hard we can't breathe
Joy

Family
My time with them is everything
Love

Disney and Universal
A different reality—filled with childlike wonder
Imagination

Concerts
The music flows through me and moves me
I swear I am invincible
Freedom

Italy
Food, culture, canals, architecture, art, cathedrals, colosseum
Beauty

NYC trips
New friends, tall buildings, inspiration everywhere
Adventure

Closed Bud

Like the lotus, I grew through dark mud and began to rise. I was ready to bloom. Well, I *thought* I was ready. My bud was still closed, but starting to open, one petal at a time. In Buddhism, a closed bud represents the time before enlightenment. I wasn't ready yet. My roots still needed the mud's nutrients for the path to full bloom.

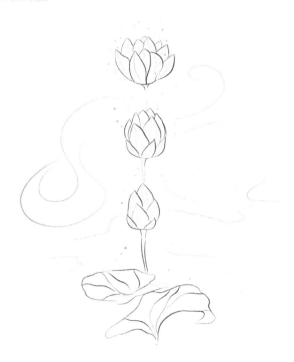

One Step Forward, Twenty Steps Back
(So it felt like)

Today started out with happiness fluttering all around me. It was a chilly October day in Northeast Pennsylvania. My absolute favorite! Today was the day Amber and I received the keys to our first apartment together. We don't officially move in until November 1st, but my uncle is our landlord, so he gave us the keys early so we could start painting and getting it ready to be a home.

This is a step into our adulthood together. Amber has been my best friend since we were five. We met in kindergarten and have been friends ever since. I was so happy to be taking this step onward together!

Before I picked up the keys, I had to do one slightly inconvenient thing. I needed a brain MRI. The other week while I was at treatment, I wasn't feeling well from a little cold I had. I mentioned a slight headache, and my oncologist immediately ordered a brain MRI. It was just one headache. I had a cold. It wasn't consistent. But he ordered it anyway.

I thought it was silly, but I still went. I worked in the morning until noon, then headed for my brain MRI. When it was over, I raced out of the clinic, went directly to my uncle's, and grabbed the keys to my new apartment.

"I heard you had a brain MRI today. How did it go?"

"Oh, fine, I guess. It was really nothing. My oncologist was just being cautious."

"Alright, well, here are your keys."

After saying goodbye to my uncle, I drove back up to Wendy's to pick up Amber. We always carpooled to work, so I told her I would pick her up as soon as she got off. I arrived early and sat in the shoe box sized break room, talking to some coworkers while I waited. I invited our friend, Christine, to join us. At the end of the shift, Amber and Christine clocked out, and we made our way to the best place in the world, Target!

We all dreamed up ways to decorate our home as we searched the place. Once we saw the prices of everything, we concluded that our dreams were too big. We were only nineteen, and it was our first apartment. We left with a few candles and an irresistible Dr. Seuss wall hanging that read, "Oh, the Places You'll Go!"

We decided to make one more stop before finally heading to the apartment. Christine wanted to go to the mall because she needed new boots for winter. When we arrived, we looked around a few stores, but our last stop was Journeys.

This is where my life came crashing down again.

I was looking at a pair of shoes when I received a call from my mom. When I answered, I heard her sobbing.

Concerned, I asked, "Mom, what's wrong?"

"You need to come home."

The only thing I could think was that something was wrong with my great-grandma. I asked, "Why? Is Gram okay?"

"Brittney, please come home. I can't tell you over the phone."

Still holding the shoe, I looked up at my friends, and they both mouthed, "Is everything okay?"

I looked down at the ground and again urged my mom to tell me.

My mom cried a moment more, then worked up the strength to mutter, "Dr. S called." She paused, then continued, "The brain MRI showed the cancer has metastasized to your brain."

That's when she lost it.

And so did I.

I dropped the shoe, hung up the phone, and fell in shock to the chair beside me.

Amber and Christine raced to my side and simultaneously asked, "Brittney, what's wrong?"

I looked up at them with a blank stare and told them I had to leave. I raced out of the store, not knowing what to do or think. My worst nightmare had just come true. I didn't feel scared yet. I felt numb. This wasn't real. Was I dreaming?

WAKE UP, BRITTNEY!! You're having a nightmare.

My friends caught up with me and begged me to tell them what was wrong. But I didn't want to. I just wanted to curl into a ball.

Still not answering them, I darted through the mall, past all the stores we just laughed and giggled in. I needed to make it to my car. I didn't know what that would solve, but I needed a safe place to collapse.

Amber caught up to me, grabbed my shoulder, and said, "Brittney! Speak to me."

In shock, I said almost too casually, "I just got a call telling me I am dying."

Amber and Christine's faces fell. "What are you talking about?" Amber asked.

"I have cancer in my brain." Saying this out loud almost sounded ridiculous. I was in disbelief.

The next thing I said was pretty harsh, but I was just so angry that this was happening again, ruining a big milestone in my life. "I guess you have to find a new roommate because I probably won't be around much longer." Once these words left my lips, I immediately wanted to take them back.

We all walked to the car in silence.

When we arrived, I gave Amber the keys and asked her to drive. I couldn't. I sat in the backseat, staring out the window, replaying the conversation repeatedly like a movie scene in my head.

"Do you still want to go to the apartment?" Amber asked, looking in the rearview mirror to get a peek at me.

"No. I don't want to see it."

"Well, where should I go?"

"Just drive around."

Then we all sat in silence, taking in the news.

Christine asked, "Is it okay if we stop at Wendy's quickly? I forgot something."

"Sure," I mumbled from the back.

I wanted to be alone, so Amber went in with Christine.

I sat in the dark parking lot alone, thinking *I'm not ready to die.*

After a while, the girls came out and asked me to get out of the car. It took some persuasion, but they finally got me out. We sat on a curb right outside of our workplace, and they both hugged me and told me they were there for me. I was so resistant to the kindness at first, but I eventually gave in and let them hold me up while I wasn't strong enough to.

"Do you want to go home to talk to your mom?" Christine asked.

"No. I am not ready." *That would make it too real.* "Let's go to the apartment."

Amber whipped out the keys, saying, "Let's go."

I sat in the back again, but we weren't silent this time. We played music, and they chatted a little bit about nothing.

When we arrived at the apartment, Amber handed me the keys so that I could do the honors of opening the door to our apartment for the first time. I took a deep breath, stuck the key in, and unlocked the door. As I turned the knob, the sadness I was waiting for punched me in the gut. A single tear ran down my cheek, and we walked inside.

As we showed Christine through all the rooms of what would soon be our home, I couldn't help but think maybe it wouldn't be. This was supposed to be a step forward, but how am I supposed to do that now?

I closed the door on what would be my room and sat down by myself. Taking long deep breaths in and out, I kneeled down into child's pose and asked God to be with me through this. "God, I am not ready to go. I still have so much life to experience. Please help me through this." I prayed. After a few minutes, I wiped the tears off my face and exited the room. The girls were downstairs, and when I got to the bottom of the staircase, I quietly said, "I'm okay." I didn't know if this was true, but I wanted it to be.

After we left, I dropped them at their homes and headed back to mine. My mom greeted me with a hug and filled me in on the plan. The next morning, bright and early, I had an appointment with a neurologist to discuss treatment.

I cried myself to sleep, hoping that tomorrow I'd be brave as I started the next chapter in my cancer journey—brain mets.

Hope Amidst Fear

I had my first neuro appointment. My mom was in denial. She demanded the doctor say it wasn't cancer. But it was. Deep down, I, too, hoped he'd say it was all a giant mistake.

Moving forward, the plan was full brain radiation. I'd start tomorrow. In the cancer world, everything is rushed. We, patients, don't even have time to digest the news we were just given. We're expected to accept our new fate immediately. I wish I'd had time to think—to fully accept—this was happening to me. I wanted to move out of fear and into faith. Unfortunately, cancer waits for no one.

My radiologist was amazing. He sent my scans to the top neurologists in the country, so they could all discuss my case. He wanted to make sure our plan was the best one. He also did this when I first met him a year and a half ago. He explained that I was young and his job was to help me live to at least eighty years old. I had a long way to go, and I was grateful he handled me with such good care.

I was scared, but I still had this tiny feeling inside telling me not to worry—that everything little thing was gonna be alright. Bob Marley, is that you? Are you in there? Just kidding.

I call this little feeling LOVE.

Mesh Mask Made for Me

I had a personalized mask made for me.
It was mesh.
It was wet.
It was warm.
And it was scary.
Is this real?
It had holes, but still,
I felt like I was suffocating.
Do I have to do this?
It started to cool
as it molded to my face.
They made some marks
and it was done.
When did this become my life?

The purpose of the mask is to help hold my head still and in the right position. It has to be exact for when I get my treatments. The making of the mask really wasn't bad. The reason for it was what I didn't like. This was not supposed to be my life.

Pleasant Surprise

As I parked my car, my phone rang. I hesitated momentarily when I saw it was my radiologist, but I answered anyway. "Hey Brittney, it's Dr. Potts. I have some really great news for you! After carefully reviewing your scans, we've decided you don't need to undergo whole brain radiation."

My heart skipped a beat. "What? Are you serious?"

"Absolutely. You're eligible for a one-day procedure called Gamma Knife, a targeted radiation therapy. This is amazing news, Brittney!"

I was overwhelmed with relief and gratitude. "Oh, my God. Thank you so much!"

"We only want the best for you. You have a long life ahead of you. I've arranged for my good friend at Penn Medicine in Philadelphia to take care of you. Someone will contact you soon to discuss the next steps and schedule an appointment."

"Okay, thank you so much," I replied, my voice shaking with emotion.

I took a deep breath and ran into the house to share the incredible news with my mom.

The Night Before

I wasn't nervous about the procedure or even so much about the side effects. I just couldn't believe this was happening. The fact that I was here, getting radiation to my brain because of cancer, was weird.

Me? Brittney Beadle with breast cancer that has barrelled to her brain. That sentence didn't even sound real.

But it was.

I didn't know what this meant for my future. My inner guidance system told me it was okay; I could handle this. I trusted and believed it, but how do I accept it?

Would this be another thing I had to live with and monitor? Would more spots pop up over the years, or was this a one-time thing?

Cancer in my body was enough to worry about but now my brain too? It felt like too bumpy and tiring of a path for one person to walk on.

No crystal ball would answer those questions for me. There was no point in focusing my energy on creating stories in my head about outcomes.

I might as well take it one step at a time.

Right now, a giant boulder blocked my way. Luckily, I was *not* alone. I could rely on the strength of my friends, family, and medical team to help me move it. If another one rolled into my path, I'd deal with it when I got to it, but right now, I had to focus on removing this one.

I believed a beautiful field of flowers was right behind it. I'd be dancing there soon.

Gamma Knife

November 15th 2016

Another early morning wake-up call for a medical procedure. We left at 2:30 a.m. to make the almost three-hour drive to Philadelphia. My dad drove while my mom and I rested our eyes.

When we arrived, they handed me paperwork to fill out and a cup to pee in. I wasn't prepared for that, so I stood by the water jug and chugged water, hoping this would help me pee. Ten minutes later, I used the bathroom and went a little.

With a reddened face, I handed it to the lady and asked, "Is this enough?"

She took it out of my hands. "Yeah, that's good."

I went and sat back down with my parents, and five minutes later, a short woman with bangs and a kind face called my name.

Smiling, she said, "Are you ready? My name is Jane, and I'll be your nurse for the day!"

"Yeah. Let's go." I said, feeling uneasy. I hugged my parents, and then we were off.

When we got down to the room, she opened a curtain, and behind it was a hospital bed. She grabbed a gown and some non-slip socks and told me to change, and she would be right back.

When she returned, she explained the game plan.

They would give me a little cocktail to make me drowsy, making it easier to place the metal frame on my head. Once the frame was on, they'd wheel me to an MRI machine—hopefully, I'd still be still knocked out. They'd get an even better look at my brain to see exactly how many lesions I had because the previous scan might not have seen them all. Once they got the results, they would determine a radiation plan, and treatment would begin.

Twenty minutes passed, and it was time for the cocktail.

The nurse walked to the side of my bed, touched my shoulder, and asked if I was ready.

I took a deep breath and nodded my head.

"Alright, here we go," she said as she started to push it through the IV.

"I am just going to close my eyes." I started counting backward in my head from one hundred. "I am starting to feel funny," I told her, and before I knew it, I was out.

I woke up in tears while they were screwing the frame on my head.

"I feel it. It hurts." I cried.

Everything after that was fuzzy because I fell back to sleep.

I woke up on a table in the MRI machine. I kept going in and out, but I remember being lifted up with a strap to be transferred back to the bed and rolled into the elevator.

When we returned to the room, the nurse came in to see how I was feeling and asked if I wanted my parents to come into the room. I said yes, and she went to get them.

When my mom walked into the room, I saw the sadness in her eyes. It must have been hard for her to see her baby girl go through this, so I cracked a joke about how I looked like a transformer. We all laughed, and it lightened the room a little bit.

The hardest part isn't the things I went through, like Gamma Knife, but seeing how it affected my loved ones.

Right before taking me back to start the procedure, my surgeon came to talk to me and tell me the plan. He told me only seven lesions were found, the size of blueberries and cherries, and the procedure would take about two hours to complete.

Shortly after, the nurse came to tell me it was time. I gave my parents one last hug, and we were off. She let me take my phone to play music during the procedure.

We entered a bare white room, cold, with no life to it. I set my phone on a nearby chair and pressed play on the music playlist I made for the procedure. Then I crawled up on the table. I scooted myself into position and slowly started to lie down with the nurse's help.

"Are you okay?"

"Yeah, I'm good," I nodded. "Let's do this!"

I felt them attach the metal frame to another piece on the table to ensure my head was completely still throughout the process. The radiation laser targeted exact spots, so it was essential I didn't move.

When we began, I just laid there visualizing my healing. Every beam not destroying but *loving* these cells into health. *This treatment is only doing good for my body.* I repeated that phrase to myself over and over again until I fully believed it.

It was a long procedure, so I dozed off, going in and out of a dream state. My dreams were pleasant and were better than my current reality. If I could, I would have stayed there a little longer, but the procedure was over, and the uncomfortable part began.

They brought me back to the bed behind the curtain and unscrewed the mask. I felt my head tighten as they unscrewed each screw one by one. It didn't hurt, but it was uncomfortable. I closed my eyes and envisioned I was on a beach with the waves hitting my knees until they were done. They then tied white gauze around my head, making me look like an awesome ninja. They said it was to protect the pin sites, where the screws were, and also for the pressure in my head.

I had a massive headache, so they gave me some Tylenol and food. The food wasn't great, but I had to eat before I could leave. They gave me a turkey and cheese sandwich, applesauce, graham crackers, chicken noodle soup, and chocolate milk. I ate a little bit of the soup and graham crackers. My dad helped me eat the sandwich, and then I was free to go.

I walked out of that hospital proud of myself and glad it was all over. I did it. It was over, and I hoped never to experience that again.

Progression

December 2016

I rested in bed all morning, clutching my fluffy blanket tightly for comfort as I waited for my oncologist to call with my scan results. I glanced at my phone every two seconds to make sure I didn't miss the call. Unfortunately, when he called, it wasn't the news I hoped for. The words "progression" and "new spots on your bones" were said.

When we hung up, I sat for a while, processing what we discussed.

No. How could this be? I only got a year out of this treatment. I was supposed to have years, remember? The doctor I saw in New York told me so. She said she has had patients alive on this since the 90s. Why didn't this work for me?

I was scheduled to start a new treatment as soon as possible, but what if it, too, didn't work? What if I ran through treatments too fast and ended up with nothing left? That couldn't happen. This one had to work. *It would work.*

And when it did, Dr. S. promised we would dance together to celebrate.

Bullshit

I tell myself if I didn't have cancer,
I would be doing *this* and *that* right now.
But because I'm sick, I can't.
I look at others who are full of health,
and I envy them.
They are so lucky.
They have more opportunities to follow their dreams than I do.

Alive

I'm still here and ALIVE.
Why am I wasting this precious time?
My future is just as important as anyone else's.

Starving

The truth is I'm not scared of dying.
I believe you never truly die; you just change form.
You leave your physical body, become pure
energy, and your soul lives on forever.

Why would I be scared of that?

What I'm truly scared of is leaving this earth too soon.
Dying before I experience everything.

I want to teach my three-year-old niece to
drive and see her graduate high school.
I want to travel to all seven continents.
I want to live by the ocean and go skinny
dipping at night in the dead of winter.

I'm starving for life, and I'm nowhere near being fed.
I will stay until I am old and gray and full of experience.

Healing Juice

Every twenty-one days, I sit my butt in a chemo chair
in a room lined with cancer patients just like me.
Well, like me, because they have cancer.
The age gap is at least forty years.

I'm used to this part of my life now, but today is a little different.
Today I sit with sweaty palms waiting on my
bloodwork to start a new treatment.

One that comes with its own set of side effects
that I will have to deal with and learn to manage.
This is the scary part of switching treatment.

I am in the unknown here.
I don't know how I will wake up feeling tomorrow
or even a week from now.

One thing I do know is
if I continue to view this treatment from a place of fear,
it won't do me any good.
So instead, I will view it from a place of love.

This treatment is going to love my cells into life.
It's going to heal and do so much good in my body.
It's going to allow me more time to live.
It's my healing juice, and I am grateful it's available.

Now let's start healing this body.

To Be Reborn
Every Morning

Every night lotus flowers submerge into murky water. The next morning they re-emerge through the mud, perfectly clean, in full bloom.

This is where my cancer loop began. Parts of me died and were reborn many times—just like a lotus flower. From this, I learned resilience. My outside environment and my body's transformation could not affect the peace within me.

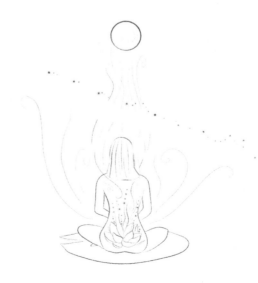

The Cycle

Starting in December 2016, I lived my life in three-month intervals—ruled by cancer.

Winter 2016/2017

December 2016 into January 2017

Despite my body's cancer progression, January's brain scan offered some much-needed relief. My scan showed the Gamma Knife was successful! All seven tumors were either gone or significantly smaller, and I was told it was still working its magic. To be honest, I wasn't surprised.

I was confident of this outcome when I went in for my scan. I had no doubt it would show healing. I just knew. Since my diagnosis, my inner gut feeling has been strong. I learned to trust it blindly, and it wasn't wrong so far.

Even though I had to navigate through new side effects from my new treatment—the biggest one being a major headache the next day that Advil couldn't touch—I chose to celebrate this win!

Spring 2017

March 2017

Two good scans! My PET showed improvement, and my MRI showed a totally clear brain! Onward to Orlando, Florida, to celebrate! If you haven't caught on, traveling to Orlando became a tradition for my mom and me after every scan, whether it offered good news or bad. This trip was a celebration! My treatment was working, and I could breathe easy for another three months.

Beach Thoughts

As I lay here on the warm beach,

toes in the soft sand,

sunshine on my face,

listening to the sounds of the waves with not a care in the world,

I realize *this* very moment is all I have.

This moment I am healthy.

This moment I am here.

This moment I am safe.

I used to really envy healthy people. They watched sunsets without thinking about how much they would miss them when they were gone. They could experience them without the conflicting emotions of happiness and sadness. Happy to witness something so beautiful but sad because they wished they had more time to take in all of this wonderful world.

But …

I slowly re-learned to release cancer from my mind. It didn't have to be present in all my thoughts. I could put it away and live just for right now. After all, I truly didn't know what the future held. No one did. I could live an entire lifetime, or I could die tomorrow from something not even cancer-related. I had no control over the timing, so why should I let it disturb my living while I am here?

Nothing is permanent.
Everyone walking this earth will die someday,
and the sun will keep shining,
the moon will still glow,
and the earth will keep spinning.
So I give my full attention to each precious, fleeting moment
because I know I'll never experience this exact moment again.

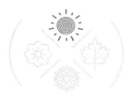

Summer 2017

May 2017

It was weird to me how fast things could change. My brain scan showed three new spots.

I had a feeling when my radiation oncologist walked in. I could tell she was about to deliver news she didn't want to. I'd learned to pick up on these kinds of cues. I always knew as soon as I saw any doctor's face. The way they'd walk in and greet me. How they'd sit down and start the conversation. It was something I could sense.

Once she sat down, she pulled up the image of my brain scan. "So," she said with a deep breath, "You do have three new spots."

Fuck. A punch to the gut.

"Do you want to see? They are very tiny, and we can do Gamma Knife again."

I leaned over in my chair to get a look at the spots. She went over each one of them with the mouse on the screen showing me where they were located and their measurements.

Yep, they're there. In my brain. Once again.

When the disappointment set in and the waterworks started, Rosie ran to my rescue by crawling up on my lap to give me a big hug. She always made me feel better.

I wasn't worried about the cancer itself because the second those words left my doctor's mouth, I felt with every fiber of my being, *It was going to be okay. Don't worry.*

I just wished I didn't have to do Gamma Knife again. The thought of the metal mask, the cold, lifeless room, the inevitable side effects, and hair loss made me shudder. I didn't want it.

I asked my doctor about full brain radiation, hoping it would eradicate the cancer once and for all. But she said there was no guarantee. It was an option, but the side effects were more severe than with targeted radiation.

After thinking about it for a hot second, I decided Gamma was the way to go.

June 5th, 2017

The scanxiety was high. The last time I had progression in my brain, I also had progression in my body. I was terrified of what my PET scan would show.

But as scared as I was, I still had a choice. Did I give in to the anxiety, or did I lead with love?

I chose to dance. I chose to surrender to what's bigger than me. I chose to love despite my current reality. I went in with faith that no matter what the scans showed, I would be okay.

Checkpoints

Sometimes it feels like there is no light at the end of the tunnel.
The treatments are forever.
Scans every two to six months.
Some days I'm so tired of it all, I wonder why I do it.
There is no finish line.

There may be no finish line. . . but I can celebrate checkpoints.

Every good scan,
every birthday,
job promotions,
anniversaries,
celebrate it all.
That's why I do it

June 6th, 2017

"Hi, Dr. S.,
Britt was wondering if
you had any news about her
PET scan?"

"It's very good. Dancing will
Happen next week!"
No Evidence of Disease

June 18th, 2017

I walked on fire. Jen hosted something called a fire walk. It's when
you walk across hot embers to break any limiting self-beliefs—like
the ones that tell you there's no way you can walk on fire because
you'll burn your feet. Many cultures have practiced this ancient
ritual.

It starts by raising your energy. Everyone gathered around the fire
in a circle. Music played, people chanted—*spirit of the fire, carry
me to my home*—drummers drummed. The fire burned bright in
the center, getting ready for us as we got ready for it.

When it was time to walk, the fire was extinguished and spread
into a flattened bed of embers. Now it was ready.

To walk on fire, I needed to extend beyond self-limitations. The firewalk was tangible proof that I was much more powerful than I realized. It was about shattering any beliefs that held me back from my highest potential. It was about quieting that inner voice that told me I wasn't enough and letting the whisper of my soul become loud and clear. *You were always enough, and you hold the power to do and accomplish your deepest desires.*

As I stepped on those hot embers, I knew in my heart I could conquer anything that came my way. Not once did I look back or stand still because I knew if I did, I would get burned. Instead, I walked straight into my future with confidence. Not a burn on my feet.

June 20th, 2017
Gamma Knife take two.

I was definitely more prepared for this go around. I knew what to expect, cocktail, attachment of the metal frame, brain MRI, radiation, and the uncomfortable feeling of removing the frame, so it was much less scary.

I had the same kind nurse, Jane, from last time. She really knew how to calm my nerves. She had a light, comforting energy about her. I guess she chose the right profession. We need more people like her in the medical field.

I woke up again mid-frame attachment but fell right back to sleep. Since my brain had only three small spots, the treatment itself was shorter. I listened to my music playlist and visualized the beams healing me again.

My current reality was weird, but I still believed I had a bright future.

Just little bumps in the road.

July 30th, 2017
Florida, my new home. I'd been making yearly trips there since before I could walk. Later in life, they became more frequent. My mom and I would fly down for a long weekend and hit Disney World and Universal Studios. After I was diagnosed, my mom, Rosie, and I took the seventeen-hour drive down almost once a month. I guess you can say we really liked it there.

I made the leap and moved over 1,000 miles away from everything I knew. I had so many fears that almost prevented me from moving. Leaving my oncologist, whom I loved, and being so far away from my friends and family—my biggest support system—wasn't an easy decision. As great as these fears were, I realized I couldn't let them run my life. Friends and family are a Facetime call away, and although I'm positive I have the greatest oncologist of all time, I'm sure there is another one who will also take great care of me. Plus, Dr. S. said he would always be there for me if I needed him.

I remember lying with Amber on our old, worn-out couch in our first apartment. We were upside down with our legs against the horrid maroon-red wall we had painted and our heads hanging off the edge of the couch, talking about life.

"One day, I am going to get out of this town. My soul wants adventure. It wants Florida." I said with stars in my eyes. "But I don't know if I have it in me to actually leave."

"You do," she said as she turned her head to look at me. "I'll miss you more than life, but it's always been your dream. It will be an adjustment at first, but eventually, it will become your home, more than this place could ever be."

She was right. A few months later, I packed up all my belongings in my car to live that dream.

Often we let fear block us, and we miss many of life's great opportunities. But I think doing the things that scare us the most is important. It shifts us out of our comfort zone so we can grow and step into the person we are meant to be.

I was so ready for this new journey in the sunshine state.

August 2017

Although I moved to Florida, I flew to Pennsylvania every two months for my brain MRIs. Changing doctors was hard. They had my life in their hands, and it took a while for me to trust someone with it fully. With my brain, I really needed someone I knew and trusted.

Going into this brain MRI, I was confident Gamma Knife had shrunk the previous spots but was nervous new ones had popped up.

When I walked into the room to discuss my results with my doctor, I knew they were good. Just like I had a sense for bad news, I also had a sense for good news. The doctor walked in cheerfully with an ear-to-ear smile on her face. She said, "Your scan was great! All three spots are gone, and no new ones!"

I jumped out of my chair and did a little silly dance to celebrate.

Once again, I had a beautiful-looking brain!

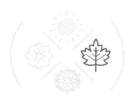

Fall 2017

October 2017
This month, I had a double WIN!

NED in the brain and the body!
I can
b r e a t h e.
But only two months later . . .

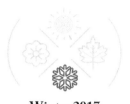

Winter 2017

December 2017
Spots.

More spots on the brain.
At this point, I honestly feel like nothing can break me.
All that is running through my mind is

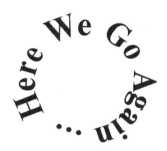

January 2018

I broke down in my doctor's office while waiting for my PET scan results. Tears shed purely from nerves.

With my knees shaking with impatience, I sat in his office, waiting for the little knock.

Every passing second felt like an eternity.

Any minute now, he will walk through with the news I want to hear!

But

What if it's what I don't want to hear? What if it's progression again?

And that's when I lost it. But instead of beating myself up over crying or being embarrassed about it when he finally did walk in, I was kind to myself. I gave myself grace because this is heavy stuff to go through.

Once again, I reminded myself it was okay to *cry*. It was okay to *feel*. It was okay to be *human*.

And the results were . . .

cue the drums ba da da da da da da . . .
Still no evidence of disease!
Hallelujah!

January 16th, 2018
"Autobots roll out!"
And just like that,
I am once again a transformer
with this metal mask
for my third round of Gamma Knife.
Third time's a charm, right?

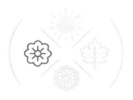

Spring 2018

April 10th, 2018
Be brave. You got this. These were my mantras every time scanxiety crept in. What a thief, stealing the inner peace I worked so hard for.

What ifs consume my thoughts, but I caught each one and fed it love.

What if there is progression turned into *I will adjust the sails.*

What if I need to switch treatment changed into *It will help my body better than this one did.*

The first step to switching thoughts was replacing them with something less scary. Sometimes my mind wouldn't let me believe positive affirmations like *I am healed* at first. I had to ease into it before I could truly believe it.

Faking a positive mindset did nothing.

Someone once told me they viewed scans as a good thing because they put you on the right path for healing. If scans showed stable, or shrinkage, or no change, it was cause for celebration. If progression appeared, you'd know it was time to try something else to put you back on the healing path.

Whatever my scans might show, I trusted all would be well.

April 26th, 2018
April not only brought the flowers, but it also brought two clear scans for my brain and body.

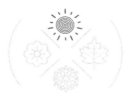

Summer 2018

May 6th, 2018

Three years. Three beautiful years of living and thriving beyond this diagnosis.

I wanted to call up that Boston doctor who gave me that time stamp of three years and proudly sing into the phone, "It's been three years, baby, and I'm still here!"

I really thought about it, but I decided it wasn't worth it. I'd become a whole new person. I had changed so much for the better and loved who I'd become. I didn't need to prove myself to anyone.

But, if I had decided to call, it would have been for everyone who got told the same expiration date as me and decided right then, and there that life was over because a doctor said so. I would have done it for them. Because they deserved better. They deserved hope. Even the smallest amount goes a long way.

July 26th, 2018

Receiving a good scan was like winning the lottery every day for the rest of your life, but ten times better. I was still NED!

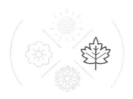

Fall 2018

November 2018
Double whammy. Again.

My PET scan showed old spots lit up and new spots lit up. The cancer was back and active. My brain also showed new spots. I needed a plan. I needed to heal. I needed to live.

November 21st, 2018
I knew I couldn't run away from my problems, but I would have been happy with a nice break from them.

I texted my good friends Vincent and Kyle to go on a road trip with me. I needed an adventure, and as always, they were down for one. Two days later, we packed up my Kia Soul and hit the road for a three-day getaway.

I loved spur-of-the-moment trips. They helped me feel free and reminded me my life was more than cancer.

We didn't have a plan which made it even more fun. We went whichever way the wind blew us.

On the first day, we stopped in Gainesville, Florida, to surprise a new friend we had recently met at an electronic dance music (EDC) festival.

We stalked his location on Snapchat maps, and we texted him to come out when we were outside. Although confused by our message, he went along with it. When he got to the bottom of the outside staircase and saw us, his jaw dropped wide open in shock. It was the best!

He generously offered to let us stay at his place for the night. We had a wonderful time together. The best part of the night was when we were driving around, and the song "I Write Sins Not Tragedies" by Panic! At the Disco came on.

It took us back to EDC when Allison Wonderland, a DJ, played it at the end of her set. We screamed the lyrics at the top of our lungs. I felt lucky to be surrounded by such great friends. I was on top of the world.

The next day we drove the rest of the way to our first destination, Atlanta, Georgia. We bundled up and explored the city on scooters, dying of laughter because Kyle didn't understand how to ride it. Every two seconds, I looked back and saw he had fallen off. Later in the day, we got the city pass and went to the Coca-Cola factory and the aquarium. We ate delicious southern BBQ and enjoyed each other's company.

The trip ended at Six Flags, where we rode all the coasters. One, we called the ball crusher because we had to stand up the entire time, and well, it crushed their balls. Never have I ever been so happy not to have balls as at that moment.

The next morning we drove back home. It was exactly what I needed, a small getaway to clear my head. A chance to live in the now.

I was ready to face whatever my future might hold.

Winter 2018

December 6th, 2018

We had a plan—kinda. I met with my oncologist, and we decided to watch the spots and not switch treatment plans just yet.

I had a small secret. I stopped taking the hormone-blocking pill without telling him. Honestly, I hated being on it. I hated that it put me in menopause at such a young age. Hot flashes are one thing, but a dry vagina? C'mon, I just turned twenty-two! I wanted a sex life. I was single and seeing someone. Having a dried-up vagina was not only painful but wasn't very sexy.

However, I confessed my secret, and I agreed to start taking it again. He said it was a crucial part of treatment. I guess sex was something else added to my plate of stuff to navigate through.

It was up to me to take care of myself so I could heal, not just my body but my mind and soul too.

December 21st, 2018
And here I am *again*.

A pig-tailed transformer about to undergo Gamma Knife for the fourth time in two years. This was metastatic breast cancer. Sometimes I had to do shitty things, but I always got through it with a smile on my face—after a good cry, of course—and a heart full of love knowing that I was okay.

Sometimes life is hard, but it is all about how you deal with it. You could choose to let it define you, or you could choose to accept it and move on. I chose the latter every single time.

December 27th, 2018

I had Gamma Knife six days ago. I felt like someone had drained every ounce of energy out of my body. I sat in my treatment chair, ready to receive the life-saving drug I knew would make me feel like I had a bad hangover when I woke up tomorrow. I felt defeated but at the same time at peace and inspired.

Sometimes life breaks you open.
If you surrender to what is
and keep moving forward,
the light will shine in.
The little break
will be worth it.
Trust the process.

February 16th, 2019

Metastatic breast cancer.
Anxiety. Fear. Uncertainty. Depression. Exhaustion. Anger.
Endless amounts of treatments.
That look on your doctor's face when you know
you are about to receive the news
that will make your soul crumble.

Metastatic breast cancer.
The cancer that has traveled
from your breast
to other parts of your body.
Incurable.

I received the news that I had more progression in my bones.
More spots on my spine, ribs, and pelvis.
I'll start a new treatment next week.
I'm not okay, but I will be.
Bob Marley echos through my entire being.
Every little thing's going to be alright.

I am in a loop with progression.
Cancer, treatment, side effects, no evidence of disease.
Cancer progresses, new treatments, new side effects, NED!
Repeat.

Excuse my language but what the fuck.

It is like I am trapped in a cave, and every time
I see a glimpse of light, I get excited.
I start running, thinking I am on my way out of here.
Then I finally reach where I thought the light was coming from,
but find more darkness.
It was all in my head.
There is no way out.

—A real experience but not the truth.

This

    Is ...

       The ...

          Part ...

             Where ...

                I ...

                   Start ...

                   To ...

                      Unravel ...

But at the same time,
I need this to happen to
break myself out of the cycle.
Sometimes things get worse
before they start to get better.
That's called healing.

Dormant, Slow Growth

In the winter months, the lotus is dormant. They stop growing and conserve their energy until next spring when the conditions are better for them to thrive. They don't die in this process. Life still spirals in its roots.

I felt dormant. I did not have ideal growing conditions. The new treatments felt like a long brutal winter, but just like the lotus, life still spiraled in my roots. Although my life appeared and even felt like it was standing still—stuck in cancerland—my roots were still alive and growing. My soul was evolving. I just couldn't see it under all the murky water.

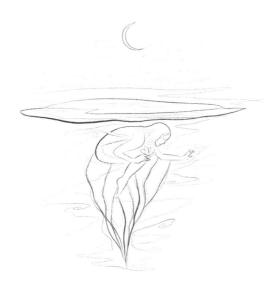

Save Me

Today I begged my oncologist to save my life.

I have a world to help change.
Please help me.
You need to save my life.

But I know deep down the only person
who can save me is myself.

Guilt of Dating

I started seeing this guy named Patrick. We met while working Halloween Horror Nights at Universal. He was *wonderful.* He moved here at the end of July from Rio De Janeiro, Brazil. He had a heavy accent which I thought was adorable. On our first date, he forgot the word "wall." He was embarrassed, but it was all part of his charm.

He had me pretty smitten. You know how people say, "When you know, you know," well, I never really believed that until I met him. The second I laid eyes on him, he drew me in like a magnet. I swear, when we locked eyes for the first time, something awakened inside of me. It was as if my soul remembered him. "Oh, there you are! I was waiting for you." It spoke.

He didn't care that I was living with cancer. I tried to hide it from him at first, well, kind of. That was before I knew him and before we went on an official date back in November. I almost made my Instagram private because I didn't want him to find out about my body's cancer. I wanted to be the one to tell him—when I was ready. Turns out, he knew long before I mentioned it, of course, from Instagram.

I guess he felt the same way about me when he first saw me. He instantly felt a connection, so he looked at the clock-in sheet at work to see my name and then searched for me on Instagram. That's how it goes with social media. All he needed was a first and last name, and he could learn everything about me in a matter of seconds.

He told me the cancer didn't steer him away from me at all. If anything, he admired me even more.

However, that was when everything was fine and dandy. Since we began seeing each other, I had progression in my brain and body. I felt *bad* for him. When we started dating, he didn't sign up to be my caregiver.

I knew it was his choice, but a piece of me still felt guilty for everything he had to go through with me. I believed wholeheartedly that I, and anyone going through this, still deserved love as much as any "normal" healthy person. Still, it wasn't easy.

Forgotten

Sometimes in life, you have to make really hard decisions.

Last week I drove an hour to my treatment center to find no plan in place and went home receiving no treatment.

This week we had a plan, so I drove an hour there again, but this time, they *forgot* to order my treatment.

I got a call telling me not to come in when I was five minutes away. How irresponsible.

I pulled into the nearest parking lot and let all my emotions flow for a good twenty minutes. Another week without treatment as the cancer is spreading.

If this were a rare occurrence, I wouldn't be so upset, but the truth is, it wasn't.

I felt constantly forgotten about and tossed to the side.

"Why didn't you look at my scans two weeks ago to have a plan set in place?" I cried to my oncologist last week when he decided to look at my results two minutes before my appointment with him.

"I just have so many patients," He said *almost* apologetically.

I didn't say anything after that. But what I wish I'd said, "But this is my life. You are holding it in your hands, and I'm counting on you. All your patients are. We are people. If you are too busy for them, maybe you shouldn't take on more than you are equipped for."

Our lives mattered even with an illness deemed incurable. When someone goes into oncology, they need much more than knowledge of the illness itself. They need patience, kindness, empathy, hope, and TIME. They are dealing with people who are falling apart daily.

Now it was my turn to make a decision. Find a new oncologist or stay?

Breath of Hope

And then some oncologists are everything I listed and more.

I hopped on the next flight and flew home to good ol' Scranton, Pennsylvania, to receive an infusion of one of my new treatments from the OG, who saved my life the first time. Dr. S.

He greeted me with a warm hug and a smile that whispered, "Everything will be okay, Brittney."

The first time around, I was bald, and he had hair. This time it's reversed. I now have a full head of golden locks, and his head is bald and shiny as can be. My oh my, how time has flown by.

Over the past few weeks, I felt like I was drowning, but talking to him was my breath of fresh air. I could breathe again. We talked about scan results, new treatments, and side effects, but as always, he ended the conversation with hope.

It's funny how I could receive good news from one oncologist and leave feeling defeated and sad but receive bad news from another and leave feeling light and having faith. That spoke volumes.

The difference in care made my "hard" decision easy. I would break up with my Florida oncologist and start seeing someone new.

Ask, and You Shall Receive

The second I surrendered and asked for guidance, the universe stepped right in. *You have to get out of your own way.*

Here's what happened. A friend told me about an alternative cancer conference about three hours from me. She suggested I message the lady who runs it and ask if I could come, so I did.

To my surprise, someone had just told her she couldn't make it and to give her ticket and hotel room—already paid for—to someone who needed it. That someone just so happened to me. Perfect timing. *Never doubt the Universe.*

But that's not all.

While at the conference, I learned amazing information from speakers from all over who healed their cancer naturally and met some fantastic people.

One was someone I knew from Instagram who I messaged when I was first diagnosed with brain mets. She is a twenty-year survivor who also had brain mets. Turned out she also lived in Orlando and told me her oncologist was taking new patients.

Shut the fuck up. *Divine timing.* I was being guided so effortlessly.

But wait, there's MORE.

My first appointment with this new oncologist went well, and we decided to take it to the next level and make it official. She is my new oncologist, and I believe I was meant to find her. She told me about a new clinical trial drug for brain metastasis. She said it looked very promising and she could get me on if I would like. My response?

HELL YEAH.

The only thing was I had to stop all other treatments until I started this new drug. Fine with me. I felt safe.

Once approved for the trial, my new treatment plan was to take the trial pill twice daily. Another chemo pill that I take in the morning and night two weeks on and one week off. This pill could also pass the blood-brain barrier. I'd get an injection to shut down my ovaries and an infusion once every three weeks.

I felt aligned and in awe of how all these events panned out effortlessly and perfectly.

Faith, Belief, Acceptance, and Trust

After Gamma Knife in December, I had a scan that showed it was successful, and all the spots healed. But my most recent scan showed two new spots.

I was offered Gamma Knife again, but turned it down.

It may sound like a crazy choice, but I'd scan again in six weeks. If the spots were still there, I promised to do radiation. I think my doctor—a new neurologist in Florida—only agreed because the trial I'd soon start crosses the blood-brain barrier.

Here's the thing. If this were anyone else, I would say do the radiation. But this was me, and for some reason, something told me I didn't need it.

After hearing about the new spots, I wasn't scared or angry and didn't wonder why this was happening again.

Before my appointment, I was reading a book called *The Science of Mind: A Philosophy, A Faith, A Way Of Life* by Ernest Holmes and read something that stuck with me.

Holmes, Ernest. *The Science of Mind: A Philosophy, A Faith, A Way Of Life* (Tarcher, Putnam, 1998)

Ernest Holmes wrote about how the body is a reflection of the mind, so for the body to heal, the mind must be at peace and there must be faith in the ability to heal. Belief, trust, and acceptance is what faith is built upon and fear is simply faith misplaced.

I decided to put my faith, belief, acceptance, and trust into both myself and something bigger than me. I would practice keeping my mind at peace. I'd observe every thought that went through my mind and every emotion I felt. Eventually, my thoughts and emotions would naturally start aligning with the future I desire—healing.

If the two tumors were still there in six weeks, I would do Gamma Knife because I believed in a beautiful mixture of the two—energy healing and modern-day medicine.

I believe in many paths to healing and that everyone has their own journey in life. I knew the risks that I was taking and the consequences that could arise. But I needed to do this. I needed to try. I didn't want to keep getting radiation every six months and also wanted to see how powerful we are as beings and if we could truly change our reality.

I was hesitant to write about this experience in my life, but I decided to because it's my truth. It was my story. It's what I lived.

I would *never* tell someone else to do the same.

What was right for me might not be right for another. Every soul has their own unique path, and I think if you get quiet, go within, and listen, you will find what is right for you

Unbound

Two months without any treatment.
I feel better than I have in a long time.

No appointments.
No treatments.
No side effects.
No chains holding me back.

I taste freedom.
It is toothsome.
I am me again.
My life is *mine*.
All mine.
Not cancer's.

How will I go back?

April 2019

I cry
And
I cry
And
I cry
Some
More

I'm talking ugly cry too.
Puffy eyes.
Snots.
Face inundated in tears.

That kinda cry as I sit in my treatment chair
receiving an infusion again.
I've started the pill form of chemo and the trial pill too.

To go from completely drug-free
to drug lockdown again is heartbreaking.
I don't know how much longer I can do this.
All my soul wants to do is fly free.

Unlimited

I wore my cute new matching green set from Aerie as I walked into my appointment. I felt confident my scan would show the spots were gone or had shrunk. I even danced in the room while waiting for the doctor to walk in.

"Where did it go?" asked my neurologist in disbelief. He zoomed into my brain scan, looking for the two spots that were there a mere six weeks ago. "It's gone! This is fantastic! The treatment must have worked fast!"

Seeing his awe-filled reaction and hearing him say, "Where did it go?" made me a little emotional. I cried *happy* tears.

I had been waiting for this moment for two years. For the past four Gamma Knife treatments, I always imagined the doctor would walk through the door in awe right before receiving the brain radiation, telling me the spots disappeared and that I didn't need treatment anymore.

Today was that day. It finally happened. My miracle.

One spot was gone entirely, and the other significantly shrunk.

I started the trial drug four weeks ago, and even if it magically worked that quickly, I think my belief in it made it work so well for me. Either way, pure energy, modern-day medicine, or a beautiful combination of both, I received my miracle. How it happened, I don't care.

I wanted to scream this news from the rooftops for all to hear! Not in a "Look at me! I healed!" kinda way, but in a "Please don't ever give up or stop believing in yourself" kinda way.

Healing is possible.

X

I haven't showered in days
Wearing the same clothes day after day
No energy, mentally or physically, to peel me out of bed
No appetite to eat a single bite of food
And if I do
I know I'll be sick
This isn't me
This isn't who I am
This is X
This is who I am on X
This isn't me
I know who I am
This is only a temporary struggle
Temporary
You hear that, X?
TEMPORARY
Please . . .
Only be temporary
I whisper as I curl up in a ball
on my messy bedroom floor
Allowing myself to cry
Cry for help
Cry to God
Cry to refresh my soul
Cry until I can't anymore

I miss myself.

Fragmented

And sometimes, you just fall and shatter
into a million little pieces.
Wishing someone could put you back together again.
Anyone, to just help you.
I have the glue and all the tools I need,
but I can't seem to use them.
I am too broken at this moment to fix the littlest piece.

Love

"Good morning, birds."
"Good morning, sun."
"Good morning, world."
"I am Brittney Beadle."
"I am healthy."
"I am strong."
"I love my life."
Patrick repeats for a second time.

"C'mon Britt, do it with me." He insists as he grabs my arm and raises it in the air.

This time we say it together, speaking it to the Universe, speaking it to my *soul*.

This is now an everyday thing. Patrick started it when he noticed my sadness. Life has been hard for me lately, but he always knows how to make me feel better.

Even if he doesn't say a word and just holds me tight.

This affirmation thing as soon as we wake up helps immensely.

It starts my day off on a light note, even though what I'm going through is heavy.

I love it, and even though I haven't told him yet, I love him.

Nightmares into Dreams

I can't sleep.
When I do fall asleep, I wake up ten minutes later.
Sometimes in a panic, thinking I'm dead.
That's the worst.
Sometimes I even forget WHO I am, total memory loss.
I jump out of bed, confused to see a man lying next to me.
I stumble while quickly putting on my clothes,
and then the memories come back,
it's my boyfriend, Patrick.
My heart pings,
and I wonder, what is going on with me?

When this happens,
I focus on my breath and
allow future visions to dance in my head.

What will it be like when I am in full health?

What will I be doing?

What thoughts will I think?

How will I feel?

Who will I *be*?

I dream it up and feel it as if this reality already exists,
then I fall asleep happily with a clear vision of my future.

I turn a nightmare into a beautiful dream,
trusting that this will be my reality soon enough.

Remember the Beauty

I'm in a constant battle with myself.
Part of me wants to live and experience life,
but the other half wishes to let go so I
wouldn't have to live like this.

Sometimes the anxiety of the scans,
fear of the unknown,
debilitating treatment side effects
are too much to handle.
I am exhausted.
This is not how I pictured my life.
The question
 Is life worth living in this condition?
enters my mind more than I would like to admit.

But then I remember.

Life *is* still worth living.

To experience fresh grass beneath my feet
marvel at the view from the mountaintop after a long climb
feel the chill of the water as I swim downriver
dance in the rain as every drip of water touches my bare skin
and to belly laugh with the people I love.

Being here on earth is worth all the heartache,
pain, sickness, and sadness.

I would do it again and again if it meant
getting to live for even a moment more in time.

The Key

Sometimes I feel as though I am stuck in a cage with a beast.
The cage is locked, and I have no key.
All I want is to wake up in the morning full of energy
after a good night's rest
and travel without being bound by
treatments and appointments.
I crave freedom from this disease.

But

Freedom is a state of mind.

My thoughts and emotions are the keys.

I can trap myself in a cage by focusing on
everything wrong with my circumstances.

Or

I can open the door and free myself
by focusing on all the beauty that still surrounds me.

I don't do well in captivity.
I break the chains of my thoughts
and bask in life's glow.

I create my reality.

The Universe responds to who I am *being*.

Love Over Fear

I was far out, deep into the ocean
all alone and full of fear.
No one could do anything to save me.
I started to drown
No sight of land anywhere.
I was losing hope fast.
Giving up seemed easier.
Let the ocean take me.
Then out of nowhere,
a feeling inside of me
told me to stop waiting for someone to save me.
It wasn't over yet.
I didn't need anyone to save me,
I needed to save myself.
I was the only one who could.

At that moment, I replaced the hopelessness with faith,
started floating instead of sinking.
I opened my heart to love,
visualized myself reaching the land.
I pictured how it would look,
how it would feel,
believed with every ounce of my being
that I would make it there.
That's when I saw it.
The land was right there

everyone I loved was waiting for me
with open arms to tell me they knew I could do it,
I just needed to believe in myself.

I swam as fast as I could and reached the land.
I was tired and worn out
but I felt great!

I looked forward to the rest of my life
because I replaced fear with love
and believed in my ability to reach shore.

The power was within me the entire time.

Goodbye X

I officially decided X isn't for me.

We tried every possible combination, two weeks on, one week off, one week on, one week off, and lowered my dose to the lowest dose possible. I still can't get past day three.

The side effects were unbearable. I felt my life draining from me more and more every day. I wasn't sure there was anything left of who I was.

I was a stranger to myself.

Maybe I could have dealt with the side effects, but I couldn't take losing myself. It wasn't worth it.

My gut told me to take myself off X, so I listened.

This didn't mean I was giving up. I stayed on my other treatments. I was determined to heal in a way that works for me. I still took control of my health and still chose what was best for my body and my life.

My oncologist wasn't happy and was reluctant to accept my decision. She urged me to reconsider. She pleaded, "We don't even know if you're receiving the trial drug, Brittney."

I told her I valued quality of life over quantity. The side effects of X were simply too much for me. With tears streaming down my cheeks, I told her, "I've given it so many chances. I want to get out of bed and enjoy life."

"But Brittney . . ." she continued.

We went back and forth with her disapproval, but at the end of the day, I knew I made the right choice for me.

I was my best healing tool. I have been all along. Health was within me; I could do this.

I choose to make decisions out of love.
Staying on X is a decision out of fear.
That is not who I am.

Lead with love, not fear.

Lead with love, not fear.

Lead with love, not fear.

Lead with love, not fear.

Lead with love, not fear.

Lead with love, not fear.

Lead with love, not fear.

Lead with love, not fear.

Lead with love, not fear.

Lead with love, not fear.

Lead with love, not fear.

Lead with love, not fear.

Lead with love, not fear.

Lead with love, not fear.

Lead with love, not fear.

Lead with love, not fear.

Unveiling the Magic

Since I was a little girl, I have always said,
"I am going to help change the world one day,"
and still, to this day, I say those exact words.

I think that's a subconscious thought that truly keeps me going.
The real reason why I'm not scared of cancer.

It's the feeling that we are much more than we think we are.

We are unlimited

perfect

whole

beings

just as we are.

We need to tap into that energy.
Then we can harness it.
Become it.

I want to be a part of helping people see the magic they have
inside of them.
It's the "purpose" I bestowed upon myself
and in the back of my mind
is always the reason why "I can't die yet."

I got things to do here, and I'm not done.

You can't change the world with an easy life.

—The truth

Reshuffle

She was dealt a bad hand of cards. She knew the deck held fifty-two. So she put the bad ones down and picked up a new hand.

Trust

It was scan day, and even though I had made decisions against normal protocols, I was feeling okay.

This was my thought process. I could put all my energy—my blind faith and trust—into the worst-case scenario. I could go down the rabbit hole of what if's trying to predict my future based on past experiences and bad scan results.

Or . . .

I could trust and believe that no matter what my scans might show, I would be okay.

If you think about it, both require energy and belief in the unknown. One just felt better than the other.

I decided to go with the latter.

All is and will be well.

Stable and Grateful

These past few months, I have taken my health into my hands.
I believe in myself more.
That's the best thing I could have ever done.

Not All Rainbows
and Sunshine

We're told to just be happy,
but sadness serves a purpose too.
No emotion is negative,
and happiness isn't a long-term destination.
It comes and goes like waves on a beach.

I think what people really search for
is peace
even in the absence of happiness.

Being content with life even on the hard days.
Knowing that even in your darkest hour,
you will experience happiness again soon.
Having joy in your heart even if you can't feel it at the moment.

So, however you are feeling, know it's okay.

Treatment Day Take 1

September 5th 2019

It was treatment day, and I was all alone for this one. I usually didn't mind going alone because it gave me time to catch up with myself and bless my beautiful body while the healing juices entered my veins to do their thing.

But today was different. Today was a long, lonely day. I arrived at 8 a.m. to do blood work and meet with my oncologist. All that went well, but now it is noon, and I still haven't started my treatment. Some days took longer than others, especially when the lab was backed up, but it never took this long.

1:00
An hour passed, and I was losing my patience. Apparently, I needed an echo before they could give me my infusion, so they are trying to schedule that. I ran through the list of everything I was grateful for and reminded myself repeatedly what an absolute privilege it was even to sit in this chair for treatment, but today it wasn't working.

2:00
I couldn't contain my emotions any longer. Waterworks rose to my eyes, wanting to fall, but I couldn't do that there. I was on the bed waiting for the technician to come in and start my echo.

2:15

She finally entered the room and set up to rub the cold jelly substance all around my heart area.

Okay, now I was really upset.

"I want you to breathe in, breathe out, then pause," she said while pushing hard on my rib cage and left breast. It took forever because she couldn't get the pictures she wanted.

Hold it in, Brittney. It's okay. It happens. Don't cry. I repeat to myself.

3:00

Done with my echo, I returned to the cancer center to receive my treatment.

3:30

Time ticked by . . . slowly . . . slowly . . .

4:00

Then I completely lost it.

I asked the nurse how much longer I had to wait before treatment started. He replied, "I'm sorry it's taking so long, but I'm not sure. They still haven't made your treatment yet."

"Okay," I replied dejectedly.

4:30

Sitting in my little chair, I began to sob. And guess what. My phone died. All hell was about to break loose.

I stomped like a child out of the room and told the nurse I'd had enough and was leaving.

"Brittney, I am sorry. Please just let me call really quickly and see how much longer. Please don't leave."

I stomped back to the chair where I sat and sobbed some more.

Ten minutes ticked by, and again I approached the nurse.

With puffy red eyes, I said, "I am really sorry, but I have to leave. I have been here for eight hours, and I am emotionally drained."

"Okay. It is going to take a little while longer, so I set up an appointment for you to come back at 8 a.m. tomorrow morning."

Though I knew better, I was acting like a child and couldn't stop. "No. I am not coming back tomorrow. I have work at 7 a.m., and there's no way I'll make it in."

Instead of fighting with me, the nurse looked at me with kind eyes and said, " Okay, but I will leave the appointment there just in case. I really hope you come tomorrow. I'm so sorry about how today went."

Man, he was so nice in the face of my wreckage. I told him, "I won't be here, but thank you."

4:45
I gathered my stuff and left with no intention of returning tomorrow.

I felt embarrassed by my behavior but understood where it came from. I didn't beat myself up over it. Honestly, I didn't think I had the energy to do so, even if I wanted to.

Treatment Day Take 2

I made it to treatment around 9:00 a.m. I knew I said I wouldn't go, but listen, I was in a horrible state of mind yesterday.

I woke up with no intention of going. My alarm went off at six. I got dressed for work and made it there at seven to clock in. But too many team members had been scheduled, so they asked if anyone would like to be on the early release list.

I am leaving this up to the Universe. I'm going to put my name on the list, and if I get the early release, I will go to treatment. I thought to myself.

About an hour later, another team member came to take my position and told me I could go home. I got an early release!

9:00

I raced out of work, not even changing my clothes, and was sitting in the little chair once again.

"Nice to see you in better spirits today, Brittney," the nurse from yesterday said.

"Yeah, I am really sorry about yesterday. I let my emotions get the best of me."

"Oh, don't worry about it. Believe me, I've seen worse." He said with that same kind smile from the day before.

9:30

My treatment was ready. They scanned the barcode on my hospital band, asked for my name and date of birth, and then started the drip.

While scrolling on Instagram, I saw my friend post that she was hosting a healing circle in Toronto in a few days. I lived in Florida, but without even thinking, I bought a ticket and told her I was coming! Being with like-minded women who want to heal their minds, bodies, and souls was exactly what I needed. This year had been tough, and I was ready to release it.

10:00

BEEP BEEP BEEP. A half-hour passed, and the signal that I was done alerted the nurses. I got de-accessed and went home to tell Patrick I was leaving for a drive to Canada the next day.

And that's exactly what I did. I hopped in my car the next morning and went to my first stop, Scranton, Pennsylvania, to see my family.

Springtime

Shorter nights and longer days.
More of the bright sun in the sky, perfect for growth.
Slowly but surely, the lotus blooms again, and so do I.

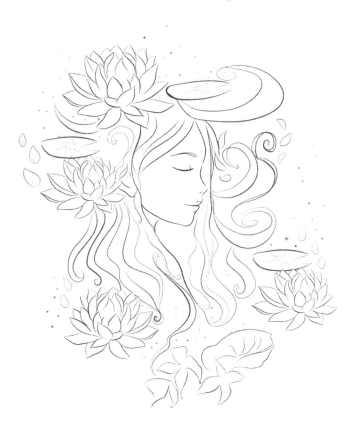

CHANGE
is
BEAUTIFUL

"The trees are about to show us how lovely
it is to let things go" —Anonymous

I let my best friend color my hair to a light brown.
I let go of the blonde that I thought I needed to be beautiful.
I cut bangs to release an old version of
me that no longer resonated.
These small changes felt freeing.

"I feel better now."

"How?

"I remembered who I am."

-A healing soul

The Release

About eighty women gathered together dressed in white. They came for one thing. Healing. Not just on a physical level but on a much deeper level. To heal the inner wounds they carried for so long.

We ate nutritious foods to nourish our bodies. We gathered in smaller groups, sharing the inner hurts, rarely, if ever, whispered. We cried and held space for one another as we did. We laughed and hugged.

We meditated, wrote down the things that no longer served us, and threw the papers into a giant cauldron. When we were ready, we all walked outside under the full moonlit sky and gathered around our two beautiful hosts as they set fire to everything we confessed—everything we wanted to release.

We surrendered. We trusted. We let go.

> —Dedicated to my Nalie Agustin, who helped me during some of my darkest days as well as thousands of others. I love and miss you every day. Until we meet again. With so much love, your Britt.

The Turning Point

What I let go of during the release

I realized something, and it sounds very messed up, but what if subconsciously, I do not want to let the cancer go? Consciously, I would do anything to be healthy and free of this disease, but when I dug deep inside, I had a realization.

All my life, I have felt worthless and like there was nothing special about me. I craved affection and to be liked by others. Then one day, I got sick, and everyone around me was there for me. I had so much attention, and I thought I did not like it, but perhaps subconsciously, I did. I was receiving so much love from everyone. It was all I ever wanted. I felt special—like I was worth something.

This is hard to admit to myself, but I think this is the "ugly" truth.

I put the ugly in quotation marks because I realize it is not ugly at all. It just is. There was a little girl who once felt alone and unwanted and manifested love in a way that was not so desirable.

I am aware of and recognize the possible block I have with releasing this disease. So now there is one thing my soul wants to do.

Dear Cancer,

You have taken so much from me, but you have also given me so much, and I am grateful for that. Thank you for showing me how to love more and not let the little things that happen get in the way of my inner peace and joy. Thank you for the amazing people I have met and the places I traveled. Thank you for my new sense of confidence. Thank you for getting me back onto the path I was always meant to walk on. I ventured off for a little while but found my way back. I think I needed you, but only temporarily. I now know my worth.

I am Brittney Beadle, and I am healthy.

I am whole.
I am worthy.
I am love
I am magical!

Thank you for coming, but I now release you!

Love, Brittney

The Sun on Our Petals

Today I danced. It was like something took over my body. There was no thinking involved, just loving movement. Beautiful music played in the background, RA MA DA SA. It was healing. It was love. It was intense in the most simple way possible. I don't know where it came from. It was right after a deep meditation. I always put on soft music afterward to get myself back into the 3D realm and to let what I had just experienced linger a little bit longer.

I have always loved to dance. Whether I'm happy, sad, frustrated, angry, scared, or whatever I feel, dancing always brings me peace and joy. At the song's end, I knelt on the floor with my hands over my heart, and I had a vision.

It was as if, in my dance, I was healing myself, and then I went on to start healing others. They then rose up to heal themselves and then moved on to help others rise and heal. It was the domino effect, but backward. We had all fallen, but then we rose again, and when we rose, we were stronger, lighter, and more beautiful than ever.

.

I believe it's time for me—time for all of us—to stop hiding in the shadows and rise into the light.

It's time for us to heal. Not just ourselves but the whole world.

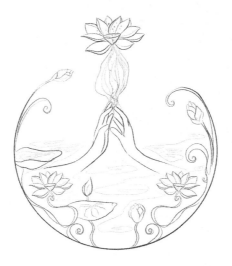

I know life is full of ups and downs, and I won't stay in full bloom forever. I'll go through the phases all over again, but each time with more wisdom to get me through. I won't stay in each phase as long as the time before, and when the sun is on me, I will cherish every little bit of it because I know it's not a permanent state of being.

I am a lotus flower.

August 2022

It's funny. As I read through this book I wrote over the years, I see the same lessons over and over again. It's a pattern I'm starting to recognize. It's as if I become a different version of myself—the person I want to be, and my body responds with healing.

It responds to who I am being. The thoughts I think, the actions I take, the feelings I feel. But when I get too comfortable, I fall back. I fall back to the person who got sick in the first place. The sad person. The old state of being. My body responds to that, and then I become sick again.

It's not my fault. Getting sick is not anyone's fault. Please never think that or feel guilty over an illness. I might be wrong. I might be right. But this is my observation about my own life.

Maybe, just maybe, this illness was my invitation to healing. An invitation to return to me. It was my medicine in a weird twisted way. It was my greatest teacher.

I am still in the midst of it all. I went three and a half years after writing this without any progression. Three and a half years. But this past year, I went through my hardest days physically. With intense bone and nerve pain and lungs covered with cancer causing shortness of breath. I started another new treatment in June of 2022. My physical symptoms are gone. No more pain, and I can breathe perfectly.

However, my scans aren't reflecting how I am feeling—yet. They show minimal response to treatment with a little progression in my bones. Still, somehow, I feel peace. A much deeper level of peace than I ever felt before.

In the past, I always felt like I had to go into "problem-solving healing mode," but not this time. Instead, I didn't feel like I had to do anything but remain in love.

I am a completely different person than the girl who wrote this book. I have experienced so much more in life. I dove deeper into my soul and learned who I am on a whole new level. I hold so much more wisdom. I used the word wisdom because I no longer have an emotional connection to what I have been through. Instead, I turned it into something beautiful.

I have absolutely no idea what my future holds. None. But I am more than okay with that. I once thought living a long life was the only option, and I wish with my entire being that's what I get to experience. But I have also made peace with the thought of death. Not in a morbid way, but in an everyone dies kind of way, and in my eyes, it's just a transition. I am okay with whatever happens, and it took a long time to get to this point. I am glad I am here.

I will live my life as intentionally as possible. I will take chances. I will allow myself to fail and succeed. I will love without limits and feel as much as I can.

I love life. I love this world, and I want to leave it a little better than I came into it. It doesn't have to be in a big way. It could just mean making a stranger smile, giving an animal a good life—like my beautiful dog Buck—helping someone in need, or inspiring someone in a rough spot. That would be enough for me.

I am learning life is simple if you let it be. Take your time, and be present with who you are now while you continue to grow. Be kind to yourself and others. Most of all, love and allow yourself to be loved.

You are worthy. Trust me on this one. You. Are. Worthy.

With lots of love,

Brittney

Gratitude

To my life partner, Patrick—I am grateful I get to know and have you in my life. Thank you for filling my life with belly laughs, inspiration, support, joy, and of course all your love. Thank you for believing in me just as much as I do and for helping to make me a stronger and better version of myself. I love you with my whole heart and soul.

To my mom, Karla- Thank you for raising me with love and magic. You are the reason I am strong enough to walk through the many challenges life has given me. You taught me to always believe in myself and miracles. I love you and I am grateful you are my mom.

To my niece, Rosie- You were so little when I went through these hardships, but somehow you always knew when I needed a hug, hand-hold, cuddle, or a laugh. We share such a special connection. I am so grateful I get to be your Aunt Britt.

To my mother-in-law, Andrea-I am beyond blessed to have you in my life. Thank you for taking me in and treating me like family from day one. You have played such a huge role in my healing journey. Saturday morning couch talks, Disney dates, cooking lessons, and all your love and support have meant so much to me.

To my soul-friend, Rachel. We share such a special connection, I swear we met a few lifetimes ago. Thank you for not only always being there for me, but also for inspiring me to go after the life of my dreams. I love you to the green planet and back.

To my very first best friend, Amber. Not many people can say they met their best friend when they were five. You are definitely stuck with me forever! You have been there every step of my journey not just with cancer, but in life. We grew up together and I hope we get to grow old together too!

To my long lost sister, Paige- Thank you for being the person I know I can always go to and receive nothing but love- also the hard truth when needed. You're a safe space for me- you know those friends that you can be your most authentic self and know you will never be judged? That's you!

To my cousin-in-heart, Hugo- Thank you for always being there to cheer me up with treats, being my workout buddy, and for your friendship. You are forever my FF!

To my good friend and mentor, Jen– You helped prepare me for what I was about to go through in life. You gave me all the tools, love, and encouragement I needed to tap into my inner power. Thank you for sharing your beautiful light with me.

To Bethany- Thank you for your help and encouragement throughout the process of writing this book and in life. I am so grateful we have crossed paths and to have you in my life!

To Dr.S- I can't even begin to express my gratitude I have for you. You were the best oncologist I ever had. You played a huge role in my healing, and not just because you were in charge of my treatments, but because you believed in me and treated me like a person, not a disease. I left every appointment, even the bad ones, feeling lighter because every conversation ended with hope. You are one of a kind. Thank you for being you.

My medical team- I want to give a huge thank you to all the amazing medical professionals who have been a part of my healing journey. I am still here today because of you. Thank you for your dedication to your patients and for your genuine compassion. You are real life superheroes.

To my soul-dog, Buck- Thank you for the joy, snuggles, and unconditional love- especially on those days where all I can do is rest on the couch.

To you, my wonderful community- Thank you for helping me feel understood and not alone. Some of my most beautiful friendships have formed because of cancer. You played a huge role in my journey whether we have talked or not. I always feel your support with me and for that I am immensely grateful.

With all my love and gratitude,

Brittney